POCKET GUIDE TO
BACH FLOWERS
ESSENCES

RACHELLE HASNAS

Certified Bach Flower Therapist

D1053848

The Crossing Press • Freedom, CA

For information on bulk purchases or group discounts for
this and other Crossing Press titles, please contact our
Special Sales Manager at 800/777-1048.

Cautionary Note: The nutritional information, recipes, and instructions
contained within this book are in no way intended as a substitute for medical
counseling. Please do not attempt self-treatment of a medical problem without consulting a qualified health practitioner.

ISBN 0-89594-865-6

Acknowledgments

I am deeply grateful to the following women, who, each in their own unique way, unknowingly have contributed to the publishing of this book: Yvonne Zahir, for bringing the Bach Flowers into my life; Karen Maresca, for her inspiring teachings of these flower essences; Lucille Arcouet, for her friendship and support, personally and professionally; Loretta Washburn Albany, dear friend and fellow writer, for her encouragement and faith in my work, and Jonnie Ruth Kuhn, my very own "earth angel," for being there for me all ways as a constant source of inspiration and love.

And my very special thanks to Linda Gunnarson, a woman of stunning vision, for making possible the further dissemination of the Bach Flower Essences with this book; to The Crossing Press publisher Elaine Goldman Gill, and her excellent editorial staff—editor Judith Pynn, for her invaluable guidance, creative insight, and extraordinary patience with a new author—and her willingness to work with my own inner vision of how this book should be, and Claudia L'Amoreaux, for her many hours of editing assistance that brought this book into its final form; to Dr. Edward Bach, for his incredible gift to humanity and the personal healing I've received from his flower essences; and most of all, I thank our Mother/Father God, for bringing the work of my heart to fruition. It's been a long road, yet, the walk has been worth it all!

Contents

For Those Who Would Heal
and For Those Who Would Be Healed

Preface

> "This system of healing...shows that it is our fears, our cares, our anxieties...that open the path to the invasion of illness...As the herbs heal our fears, our anxieties, our worries, our faults and our failing...then the disease, no matter what it is, will leave us."
>
> Dr. Edward Bach

It is a great honor and pleasure for me to share with you this information on the Bach Flower Essences. I was first introduced to the Bach Flowers in 1987. It's hard to believe that almost ten years have passed! When I first began my education and training in this extraordinary self-help system that Dr. Bach developed, little did I know then that I'd be bringing his work to so many others.

For years I had been interested in holistic healing, exploring many alternative techniques for facilitating the healing process. When the Bach Flowers came into my life, I knew I had found a healing modality that was truly exceptional. Over these many years, the flower essences have been a catalyst for personal growth and emotional healing in so many areas of my own life. And as a Certified Bach Flower practitioner, I have been witness to many remarkable transformations facilitated by the flower essences for those I've counseled.

I soon discovered I had a mission—a deep desire to share Dr. Bach's gentle healing gifts of nature with as many people as possible. In 1995, I was given the opportunity to do this. It has been my privilege for almost two years now to present extensive programs on the Bach Flowers in many parts of the country. And now I have been given the awesome opportunity to again share the Bach Flowers—with the publishing of this book.

It is my greatest hope that after reading about the Bach Flower Essences and actual case studies illustrating their efficacy, you will go on to discover for yourself, what I have.

Once you have experienced their gentle, yet profound healing power, I am confident your life will never be the same! Not only will you be using the Bach Flower Essences for yourself, but you will be also teaching others.

"And may we ever have joy and gratitude in our hearts that the Great Creator of all things, in His Love for us, has placed the herbs in the field for our healing."

Dr. Edward Bach

Dr. Edward Bach and His Philosophy of Healing

"We each have a Divine mission in this world, and our souls use our minds and bodies as instruments to do this work, so that when all three are working in unison the result is perfect health and perfect happiness."

Dr. Edward Bach

The Bach Flower Essences were developed in England in the late 1920s and early 1930s, by renowned British researcher and physician, Dr. Edward Bach. They are considered the first in what is now considered vibrational medicine. Bach, a brilliant physician, bacteriologist, immunologist, and pathologist, eventually turned from the orthodox medicine of his day to that of homeopathy. It was his understanding that to truly cure disease, the treatment of symptoms was not adequate. One needed to get to the root cause of disease for any cure to be lasting.

It was Dr. Bach's belief that a negative state of mind was at the core of any illness. It was not enough for him to treat the body alone. Body, mind, and spirit all needed to be considered in regard to healing. He was concerned about the treatment of the whole person. It became his dream to develop an entirely new system of medicine based upon his insight. He soon gave up his lucrative medical practice and began his search which took him back to the English countryside. He intuitively knew that there, among the flowers and trees of the field, he would find the healing properties that he was seeking.

One morning, while walking through a meadow, his highly developed sense of intuition made him realize that the dew on the plants, heated by the sun, now held the healing properties of the flowers it laid upon. As he continued his work, his intuition became so sensitive that, by holding a flower or tasting a petal, he could immediately sense what its healing effects were. In this way, one by one, he found and developed the 38 different flower essences that have come to be known today as the Bach Flower Essences.

Dr. Bach was a deeply spiritual man. His philosophy about disease was tied into his philosophy about life. He wrote in *Ye Suffer From Yourselves*, "Disease of the body, as we know it, is a result, an end product of something much deeper. Disease originates above the physical plane, nearer to the mental. It is entirely a result of a conflict between our spiritual and mortal selves. So long as these two are in harmony, we are in perfect health: but when there is discord there follows what we know as disease."

It was Dr. Bach's belief that we are more than physical beings—we are spiritual beings in truth, each coming into this world with a certain purpose or mission to fulfill. When we become out of sync with our spiritual purpose, disharmony arises. This can come about by interference of other people—allowing them to push us off our course—or by our own moods, fears, or hesitations. Dr. Bach further wrote in *Ye Suffer from Yourselves*, "Whatever errors we make, it reacts upon ourselves, causing us unhappiness, discomfort, or suffering…The object being to teach us the harmful effect of wrong action or thought: and by its producing similar results upon ourselves, shows us how it causes distress to others, and is contrary to the Great and Divine Law of Love and Unity."

As we can see from his writings, he considered disease beneficent and purely corrective—a message from our soul that changes need to occur in our lives if we are to find and maintain our health and happiness. He goes on to write that disease "is the means adopted by our own Souls to point out to us our faults: to prevent our making greater errors: to hinder us from doing more harm: and to bring us back to the path of Truth and Light from which we should never have strayed."

It was his contention that in order for health to exist, there must be perfect harmony between body, mind, and spirit. And it was this harmony alone that needed to be re-established for any lasting cure to be effected. To this end he developed the flower essences—to release the emotional and mental disharmony within us, to facilitate being true to our soul's purpose once again, thereby restoring our system's equilibrium. As he wrote in *The Twelve Healers and Four Helpers*, "It is not possible for us to be ill unless we are not in harmony with our true nature. But whatever condition is behind our trouble, whatever fault there is in our nature it matters not, because these remedies will help us to correct that fault and thus curing the root-cause of our illness and give back to us bodily and mental health."

Thus it would seem from Dr. Bach's writings that the presence of germs, or even our genetic make-up, although they may play some part in the development of illness, are not the true cause of lack of health. This is a profound insight and one that brings to us a whole new way of looking at health and healing.

Dr. Bach wrote, "These [negative states of mind], if we allow them, will reflect themselves in the body causing what we call disease. Not understanding the real causes we have attributed disharmony to external influences, germs, cold, heat, and have given names to the results, arthritis, cancer, asthma, etc.: thinking that disease begins in the physical body."

The old model of looking at the human body as merely a machine may be on the verge of extinction—and long overdue. Our materialistic view of life is being challenged with the recognition of a spiritual component that has, for too long, been overlooked. We are living in exciting times!

Bach Flower
Essences Defined

You are about to begin a sacred journey, a journey of self discovery…one that opens you to personal growth and emotional healing. I'll be sharing with you concise information on Dr. Bach's flower essences—their use and effect—gleaned from my personal and professional experience, to give you a deeper and richer understanding of the energy in each and to facilitate your selection of the appropriate flower essences with confidence.

You'll soon learn how the flower essences can assist you in just about any area of your life where you find yourself emotionally out-of-balance. When you're having difficulty in coping with the situations you face in these stress-producing times—whether it's worries and fears, lack of self-esteem, or even depression, the flower essences can help. And as we are now beginning to recognize, these negative emotional states may be the catalysts to the eventual development of disease.

It is interesting and exciting to note that traditional Western medicine is now taking notice of the mind-body connection, and beginning to recognize that emotions play a much greater role in the body's health than was believed or understood before. For several years now, studies by psychoneuroimmunologists are being conducted in leading universities and research centers countrywide, establishing a firm link between the mind, emotions, and the body. It has now been proven that negative emotions do have an ill effect on our well-being. Psychoneuroimmunology is a relatively new branch of medicine which has been studying brain chemistry in relation to stress. It appears from these studies that adverse neurotransmitters are produced by the brain when we are under stress, deleteriously affecting the immune system, our body's first defense against disease. The longer this biological process continues unchecked, the more vulnerable we become to the onset of any number of disorders.

We know that high blood pressure, ulcers, migraine headaches, heart disease, allergies, and asthma have all been linked to stress. As far back as May 24, 1983, this link was reported in an article in *The New York Times* entitled, "Emotions Bound To Influence Nearly Every Human Ailment." It stated, "virtually every ill that can befall the human body—from the common cold to cancer and heart disease—can be influenced, positively or negatively, by a person's mental state." It appears that Dr. Bach was well ahead of his time, with modern medicine only now catching up!

Before we explore the 38 Bach Flower Essences in depth, a short introduction to what they are and how they work is needed for those not familiar with them.

Please remember, the flower essences are an adjunct modality to be used along with traditional medical treatment. They work as catalysts in restoring and balancing your body's own healing system.

SIMPLICITY, HUMILITY, COMPASSION

These three words are inscribed on the plaque which hangs over the door of the Bach Center in England. They are more than just words acknowledging Dr. Bach's contributions to humankind. They also have a powerful message for all who are open to hear. The flower essences can teach you the true meaning of these words, as they assist in bringing inner peace and a sense of well-being into your life.

Simplicity—The flower essences teach us that things don't have to be complicated. These natural preparations, carefully made from the essences of flowering plants, offer a complete, effective, safe, yet simple system of gentle stress relief—a system that allows you to be involved in your own healing process. It was Dr. Bach's intention that his system be so safe and simple that anyone could use it at any time, even during pregnancy. To paraphrase his words, he wanted it to be so simple that when an individual was hungry they would go to the garden and pick some lettuce, and when they were afraid they'd take a dose of Mimulus (one of the 38 flower essences he developed to counteract known fears).

Humility—As you begin selecting your flower essences, you'll find as I have, that this is a journey of self-discovery, for you are learning about the personal issues and conflicts inside yourself that are the cause of disharmony within you. Humility becomes crucial, for it allows you to be open to self-reflection which ultimately can lead to personal growth. To be honest with yourself and admit that change may be needed takes great courage and strength. Yet this is a necessary step on your journey to wholeness. By looking within and being in touch with your feelings, recognizing your negative states of mind, you'll better able to select the essences that relate to you. You will understand the issues that have been holding you back from living life in a richer, more meaningful way.

Compassion—Dr. Bach's flower essences were developed out of his love and compassion for humanity. He felt a calling, even as a young boy, to be able to help people heal. As you work with the flower essences personally, you'll find yourself recognizing certain flower essences that could be helpful to others you know. You will begin to see the flower essences, not only as facilitators of change in your own life, but as special gifts to be shared from your deepening sense of love and compassion, as did Dr. Bach.

The Bach Flower Essences contain certain properties taken from 38 specific flowering plants and trees that Dr. Bach determined to have special healing attributes, with the addition of pure spring water and brandy, added as a preservative. Like other natural medicine, they take effect through treating the *whole* individual, not the disease or symptoms of disease. Therefore, they are *never* selected for any specific symptom or condition. The negative emotional state determines the selection.

As an example, two people, each with the same disease—perhaps high blood pressure—would more than likely each benefit from a different flower essence. One may have developed the condition because of an impatient nature, the other from an overly critical one. Hence, a different flower essence, with its unique vibration, would be appropriate for each individual. The person who is overly critical, and takes the Beech flower essence for this state of mind, would experience increased tolerance. The individual who is impatient, and takes the Impatiens flower essence for this state of mind, would experience more patience. Their own potential for self-healing will be reinstated, freeing the physical system of the stress that was originally creating these conditions.

In the cases of these two individuals the flower essences were selected for their particular negative emotional states. They were *not* chosen for their symptoms or conditions. The Bach Flower Essences work by transforming (rather than suppressing) negative attitudes or emotions into positive ones.

The Bach Flower Essences are a form of energetic or vibrational medicine, as it is now termed. The energy or vibration taken from the flowers gently affects and enhances our system on subtle levels. In *Vibrational Medicine*, Dr. Richard Gerber defines this energy medicine as "That healing philosophy which aims to treat the whole person—the mind/body/spirit complex—by delivering measured quanta of frequency-specific energy to the human multi-dimensional system. Vibrational medicine seeks to heal the physical body by integrating and balancing the higher energetic systems which create the physical/cellular patterns of manifestation...Vibrational medicine is a healing approach which is based upon the Einsteinian concept of matter as energy, and of human beings as a series of complex energy fields in dynamic equilibrium."

With his great sensitivity, Dr. Bach was also aware that we have a series of energy bodies within our physical body. He wrote in *Heal Thyself* that, "Materialism forgets that there is a factor above the physical plane which in the ordinary course of life protects or renders susceptible any particular individual with regard to disease, of whatever nature it may be. Fear, by its depressing effect on our mentality, thus causes disharmony in our physical and magnetic bodies and paves the way for (bacterial) invasion. The real cause of disease lies in our own personality...."

The flower essences were created to work on these subtle bodies, for it is here where our system's equilibrium has been disturbed by our negative attitudes and emotions, with the mind-body connection coming into play. And it is here where the flower essences can balance and restore our system's homeostasis once again.

As you go through your selection process, remember to choose your flower essences solely with regard to the out-of-balance emotional or mental states you may be suffering from—such as impatience and being overcritical. There are many other stress-producing emotions that the Bach Flower Essences bring balance to, such as fear, bitterness, lack of self-esteem, denial or repression, resentment, apathy, guilt, to highlight several more. Dr. Bach felt that *all* known negative emotional states are addressed by them and considered his flower essences a *complete* system.

It cannot be emphasized too strongly that Dr. Bach believed that it was our negative states of mind that were the root cause—the very breeding ground of disease—and, if left unchecked, the catalyst for eventual illness and symptom manifestation. Dr. Bach wrote, in *Free Thyself,* "This disharmony, disease, makes itself manifest in the body for the body merely serves to reflect the workings of the soul; just as the face reflects happiness by smiles, or temper by frowns. And so in bigger things; the body will reflect the true causes of disease (which are such as fear, indecision, doubts, etc.) in the disarrangement of its systems and tissues."

By selecting the appropriate flower essence that remedies the particular negative emotion, the healing properties contained in the essence act like an antidote. A flower essence has the ability to gently and safely release negative emotional states by flooding the body's system with the positive vibration it carries. Over time, emotional balance is again restored. It is important to state again that the flower essences *never* repress emotional imbalances. Rather, they are catalysts for their release.

The flower essences don't have the effect of tranquilizers or antidepressants, aren't considered herbs or vitamins, and won't interfere with the effects of other medication being used. Because the flower essences are so safe and gentle, you cannot overdose in their use. Dr. Bach's self-help system is totally safe, natural, and harmless, without need for any concern over the possibility of side effects. And when kept in a cool, dark place, the flower essences have an indefinite shelf life. As this system of healing is a very individualized modality; there is no specific length of time as to how long you need to take them. Many flower essence users report that they feel the effects within two to six weeks. Individual sensitivity is a factor here; thus, the reaction time is different for each individual.

Know that a commitment to the flowers essences is important for them to be effective. If you are not committed to using them consistently , you'll think they don't work. Most flower essences need to be taken from one to two months. Only you can determine when your issues have been released. If you stop too soon, and your issues reappear, just continue to take them for a while longer. Another factor in your reaction time to flower essence use is how long you have been dealing with a particular emotion or issue, and how deeply ingrained into the personality it has become. The more deeply ingrained, the longer will be the reaction time.

The question of the Bach Flower Essences being a placebo comes up many times. This placebo effect has long been an accepted phenomenon in medical practice, although little understood. The answer to this question is a definite no. It is not just mind over matter that produces the flower essences' positive effects. A placebo study was done by Michael Weisglass, Ph.D. at the California Institute of Asian Studies in 1979. His study showed the flower essences to have a much greater effect on those who actually took them, in comparison to the control group—those who were not given the flower essences, but only thought they were taking them. In his research he found that the flower essences operated independently of the belief system of the user.

Young children and animals have no awareness that they are being given any special medicine to bring about any emotionally related changes. In my work with them I have found the flower essences to indeed have a marked effect in bringing about relief. This will be further illustrated with case studies in later chapters on the use of the flower essences with children and animals.

The next chapter will assist you in identifying the flower essences you may need. The indications which describe the out-of-balance emotional state(s) and/or personality trait(s) that each flower essence addresses are clearly and simply presented. As you read through this information, it is suggested to keep paper and pen handy to make note of which flower essences speak to you. Choose the ones that relate to your specific emotional issues and character traits that cause you problems.

It is recommended that no more than seven flower essences be used at any one time. It is not unusual at first to find yourself feeling you could use almost all of them. The key to limiting your selection to only seven is to focus on the issues that are the most intense for you right now—the ones that cause you stress on a daily basis. Of course, it's important to choose the appropriate flower essences to benefit from their effects. However, it is also reassuring to know that no harm can be done if you make a wrong selection. In this case, nothing happens. You will only respond to those that you need.

THE BACH FLOWER ESSENCES—
KEYWORD INDICATIONS

KEYWORD INDICATIONS CONTINUED

The Bach Flower Essences	Keyword Indication(s)	Page
Mustard	sudden depression	43
Oak	bravely endure all obstacles	44
Olive	extreme exhaustion	45
Pine	perfectionism, self-blame, guilt	46
Red Chestnut	overconcern, anxiety for others	47
Rock Rose	panic, terror	48
Rock Water	self-denial	49
Scleranthus	indecision, vacillation	50
Star of Bethlehem	grief, shock, trauma	50
Sweet Chestnut	extreme mental anguish	51
Vervain	overenthusiastic, opinionated	52
Vine	domineering, inflexible	53
Walnut	easily influenced by others	54
Water Violet	aloof, proud	56
White Chestnut	obsessive thoughts, restless mind	57
Wild Oat	uncertain of path in life	58
Wild Rose	apathy, resignation	59
Willow	bitterness, resentment	60

Indications for the 38 Bach Flowers

1–AGRIMONY

Botanical Name—*Agrimonia Eupatoria*
Vibration—*joyfulness*

Indications: Agrimony is indicated for those who do not acknowledge their feelings of pain and torment, but repress and deny their feelings, putting on a brave front, a cheerful facade. "Everything's fine," they say. Many times these individuals turn to alcohol or drugs to help mask feelings that are too difficult to face. Be aware, however, that substance abuse does not always have to be a part of the Agrimony personality to indicate the need for this flower essence. Other avoidance techniques can come into play: an addiction to TV as in the couch potato syndrome, overeating to numb emotional pain, as well as any other activity to ensure the repression of feelings. The Agrimony Type is driven to avoid torments at all costs. They shy away from confrontations and arguments, needing to keep the peace at any price.

Agrimony is suggested for use when in counseling, as it facilitates openness in getting in touch with what has been repressed or denied and releases buried issues, allowing emotional healing to take place.

Examples: This flower essence profile relates very much to the personality of Marilyn Monroe. Some other well known personalities that reflect the Agrimony profile are the TV character from *All in the Family*, Edith Bunker, who always seemed to be in denial regarding her feelings, and TV news anchorwoman, Jessica Savitch, who died in an automobile accident. Since her death it has been revealed that her personal life was filled with deep emotional torment. She turned to drugs and alcohol to ease her pain.

2–ASPEN

Botanical Name—*Populus Tremula*
Vibration—*fearlessness*

Indications: This flower essence, one of several available for treating states of fear, is indicated when the source of fear is *unknown*, such as with feelings of foreboding, uneasiness, apprehension. Use it when you don't really know what it is you're afraid of, yet you are experiencing feelings of fear. Nightmares, fear of the dark, and sometimes even a fear of God or the supernatural can bring on the Aspen state. Anxiety and panic attacks are also states that are relieved by this flower essence. The mark of the Aspen profile is the inability to put your finger on exactly what it is that is causing your fear, anxiety, or apprehension—the source being very vague and unclear.

Examples: The form of fear that Ebenezer Scrooge experienced with the appearance of the ghosts of Christmas past, present, and future in Dickens' *A Christmas Carol*, describes a facet of the Aspen state perfectly.

3–BEECH

Botanical Name—*Fagus Sylvatica*
Vibration—*tolerance*

Indications: The indications for this flower essence are extreme criticism and intolerance of others—constant fault finding and judging. In most instances, feelings of intolerance are verbalized, but this doesn't have to be the case. The Beech Type may just observe and ruminate at how annoying others seem to be. There's a constant condemnation concerning others when in the negative Beech state. One is unable to accept others as they are. This flower essence is indicated for those with intolerance, as well as feelings of prejudice towards others—being judgmental to the extreme.

Examples: Jesus exemplified for us the most positive aspect of the Beech state, when he uttered, "Father forgive them, for they know not what they do." Felix Unger, the movie and TV character from *The Odd Couple*, is a perfect example of the out of balance state that Beech addresses, with his constant criticism of roommate Oscar. The comedians Don Rickles and Joan Rivers, and not to forget Carroll O'Connor in his role as Archie Bunker from TV's *All in the Family*, all beautifully portray the negative Beech state in their performances. By the way, Beech is the perfect flower essence to take before going to a family reunion—both for dealing with the possible intolerance of your relatives, and their possible intolerance of you!

4–CENTAURY

Botanical Name—*Centaurium Umbellatum*
Vibration—*self-determination*

Indications: In the negative Centaury state, the ability to refuse others' requests is difficult, if not impossible. These people are easily taken advantage of. The desire to serve others is really an admirable attribute although not when it is constantly at one's own expense. Being a doormat is not healthy. In fact, resentment develops when personal needs are always put aside. Centaury Types find it hard to let others know they are feeling resentful, and continue to allow others to use them. This cycle will persist, creating even greater resentment. They will hurt themselves in the process with the underlying negative emotions that result. Centaury Types don't like to make waves, to displease others, to be disliked; they find it extremely difficult to stand up for themselves. This behavior is classic co-dependency, and many have found Centaury helpful in releasing their victim issues.

It is as important that each of us is able to take care of ourselves, as it is to serve and help others. This is the lesson of the Centaury state. When giving to others is detrimental to their own welfare, this flower essence enables individuals to be able to say, "No—I'm really sorry, I'd love to help you out, but it's not possible now—maybe another time." Centaury allows us to do this gently and feel OK with it and know, "I can do what I need for myself. I don't always have to sacrifice my needs for others." We each need to learn to honor the spirit in us, as well as in others. It is our right and duty, actually, to consider and take care of ourselves. If we cannot love and nurture ourselves, how can we honestly love and nurture anyone else truly from our hearts? Dr. Bach indicated that Centaury Types are on the road to being of great service—although their motives are good, they are being passively used instead of actively choosing their own work.

Examples: When I think of the indications for Centaury, Cinderella always comes to mind. This fairy tale character is really the perfect example of the Centaury profile— always willing to please others at her own expense—always willing to serve and never say NO. Again, we turn to Edith Bunker, portrayed by Jean Stapleton, as an excellent illustration for the Centaury profile, always putting her own needs last, if considering them at all.

5–CERATO

Botanical Name—*Ceratostigma Willmottiana*
Vibration—*inner certainty*

Indications: The indication for this flower essence is an extreme lack of self-confidence in decision making, which leads to constant dependency on others' advice. "I need to make a decision, but I don't have enough confidence in myself. I'd better check with Mary and John, also Sally and Jim, and find out what they think I should do." Cerato people check it out, they are told what to do and then maybe a day or two later, realize that the advice was wrong and they should have gone with their own feelings, after all. Cerato is indicated for those who lack confidence in their own judgment—always seeking advice and reassurance from others before they can act. Cerato releases this deep-seated reliance on others, bringing an inner confidence and ability to rely on one's own discernment. This Type is exemplified by the psychic junkie—always going from one consultation to the next, looking for answers that really lie within.

Examples: Kirstie Alley's portrayal of Rebecca in the TV show, *Cheers*, illustrates the Cerato profile, with Rebecca always going to the rest of the characters for advice.

6–CHERRY PLUM

Botanical Name—*Prunus Cerasifera*
Vibration—*composure*

Indications: This flower essence addresses the fear of losing control in some way. These Types wish to harm themselves or others by taking unneeded risks or acting rashly. Cherry Plum aids in restoring self-control and helps bring an awareness of what's really in one's best interest. It is highly recommended in times of extreme emotional crisis, when there is danger or threat of suicide. There are many other situations—or Cherry Plum states—where there is a tendency to lose control, such as in temper outbursts, abusive behavior towards others, out-of-control gambling, and credit card use, as well as substance abuse. In fact, Cherry Plum is helpful for risk taking of all sorts. It has also been extremely successful in treating obsessive-compulsive behavior.

Examples: Kurt Cobain of the rock band Nirvana was in an extreme Cherry Plum state when he committed suicide. Musicians Janis Joplin and Jimi Hendrix, with their history of substance abuse and loss of control, are other examples of Cherry Plum Types who are out of balance.

7–CHESTNUT BUD

Botanical Name—*Aesculus Hippocastanum*
Vibration—*capacity for learning*

Indications: Chestnut Bud would be indicated for those who do not seem to learn from past mistakes, and continue to repeat the same old habit patterns that cause difficulty for them. In this state there seems to be a lack of observation. As an example, let's take a situation in which Chestnut Bud would be indicated. In this case scenario, an individual is constantly attracting unhealthy partners many times over— perhaps an alcoholic, or abuser. Each time the dysfunctional relationship is ended, like magic, the identical personality type, with a different name of course, appears at the doorstep, and once again, is invited in! Old patterns are hard to break. However, when you are ready to face the destruction they cause you, Chestnut Bud is waiting to help you learn from the past and act with more wisdom in the present. This flower essence is also highly recommended in releasing addictive behaviors.

Examples: Jerry Garcia, from the Grateful Dead Rock Band, would exemplify the out of balance state with his on again, off again use of drugs which eventually destroyed his health and led to his death. Nicole Simpson is another illustration of the Chestnut Bud profile, returning several times to an abusive relationship.

8–CHICORY

Botanical Name—*Cichorium Intybus*
Vibration—*selfless love*

Indications: The indications for this flower essence are represented perfectly by those who exhibit the Mother Hen syndrome—the over-possessive, over-nurturing types—female or male—who tend to smother those they love, as well as want absolute control over their lives. They can also be martyrs but expect to be rewarded for any perceived sacrifice, and will be filled with self-pity if none comes. They are often heard to say, "And after all I've done for you, this is how you treat me!" The love they so generously give has invisible strings. They are possessive, self-centered, and demanding in their strong need for attention and appreciation, and are not above manipulation to get what they want. The Chicory Type, once in balance, gives love freely, no longer requiring anything in return.

Examples: The character Cliff (the mailman), from the *Cheers* TV show, had a mother who portrayed the Chicory profile to a "T," with her constant need for attention and manipulation of her son.

9–CLEMATIS

Botanical Name—*Clematis Vitalba*
Vibration—*creative idealism*

Indications: The profile for the out of balance state this flower essence treats is that of excessive daydreaming and lack of concentration. The Clematis Type appears to be lost in another world, and finds it hard to be in the here and now.

Dr. Bach called Clematis the flower essence for "polite suicide," as he felt these individuals had lost interest in daily living, letting life simply slip by. In the Clematis state, there is a strong need to escape from life on some level. Preoccupied with their fantasy worlds, these individuals are not really happy with their lives. Yet, they take no action to create change for themselves. These people are often highly artistic, but lack the ability to express their gifts in practical and material ways. They tend to lack energy and appear listless, and are often drowsy during the day. They would rather be alone, do not like confrontation, and avoid this by withdrawing. Clematis is highly recommended for grounding—to bring focus to the present and to encourage taking an active role in life. For many children with learning disabilities, Clematis is frequently used with great success.

Examples: For those familiar with the fictional character Don Quixote, it is easy to recognize the out of balance Clematis state he personified. Rip Van Winkle is another character who was, without doubt, in the Clematis state!

10–CRAB APPLE

Botanical Name—*Malus Sylvestris*
Vibration—*purity*

Indications: Crab Apple is the flower essence for cleansing. It is also indicated for those who feel unclean, or dissatisfied with their body image. There may even be feelings of self-disgust regarding the body. Crab Apple Types don't accept themselves as they are, many times blowing out of proportion a particular physical flaw they perceive they have—"My nose is too long, I'm too fat, my hair is too thin," and the list goes on.

Crab Apple can be extremely helpful in treating anorexia and bulimia, as those who suffer from these conditions have an obsession with their weight. This flower essence is also a great help for women during the end stages of pregnancy, when they look in the mirror thinking, "my God, I look like a beached whale. Where did that waist line go?" As Crab Apple is a cleanser, it is also recommended for pregnancy in general, as the body is now cleansing two life systems.

In cases of rape and incest, Crab Apple is indicated, as these victims experience feelings of being soiled and unclean. Crab Apple assists in releasing the toxic emotions of shame, guilt, self-loathing and disgust, so as to pave the way for the process of emotional healing to begin.

Examples: Again, we look to Felix Unger, the character from the movie and TV show, *The Odd Couple*, who is also an excellent example of the out of balance Crab Apple state. His name should be Mr. Meticulous! It would also seem he was a bit obsessive about his health with the nose spray, and his extreme concern for dirt and germs.

Michael Jackson is an extreme example of the Crab Apple Type with his obsessive concern for his appearance.

Millionaire Howard Hughes also exemplified the Crab Apple profile to the *n*th degree. Towards the end of his life he became obsessive-compulsive over germs to such an extent that anyone or anything entering his home had to be sterilized!

Princess Diana is another illustration of the Crab Apple state, with her reported past struggle with anorexia.

11–ELM

Botanical Name—*Ulmus Procera*
Vibration—*right responsibility*

Indications: The negative Elm state is usually temporary. It comes about when there is too much to do and not enough time or energy available to do it, and the feeling of being over-whelmed is experienced. This state usually affects responsible people who normally are able to handle their affairs. When our plate becomes too full, quite suddenly we may experience exhaustion, and feel overwhelmed and inadequate to handle everything. The flower essence Elm brings a confidence that you can accomplish all you need to, in the right time and place.

Examples: The nursery rhyme character, The Old Woman Who Lived in a Shoe (and had so many children she didn't know what to do!) is a prime example of the Elm state!

12–GENTIAN

Botanical Name—*Gentiana Amarella*
Vibration—*faith*

Indications: The indications for this flower essence are feelings of despondency that come with setbacks and delays— with situations not going as planned. "Why can't things ever go right?" you wonder. The out of balance Gentian state is a "what's the use, anyway" kind of feeling. When this occurs often enough, one begins to feel tired and depressed, with a loss of faith. For these feelings of discouragement due to life's inevitable setbacks and delays, Gentian seems to melt away those negative feelings. It brings a knowing that it will eventually work out. In most instances in life, we have very little control over the progress of a situation. Once we've done our part, we need to let it run its course as it will, and not allow ourselves to be unduly discouraged. We need to keep the faith that all is indeed working in divine order! This flower essence also aids children with learning disabilities, as their progress in school, many times, is a struggle, often producing feelings of discouragement and failure.

Examples: The Hunchback of Notre Dame portrays this state so poignantly; the constant setbacks in his life created discouragement and frustration for this poor soul.

13–GORSE

Botanical Name—*Ulex Europaeus*
Vibration—*hope*

Indications: Dr. Bach noted that Gorse individuals looked as if they needed sunshine in their lives. The indications for the Gorse state are feelings of hopelessness and extreme despair. One feels as though nothing more can be done. The feelings experienced here are deeper and more pervasive than in the Gentian state.

Examples: We can look to Shakespeare's *Romeo and Juliet* for the most definitive portrayal of this state. Both these lovers went into such a state of hopelessness, they chose to end their very lives.

14–HEATHER

Botanical Name—*Calluna Vulgaris*
Vibration—*empathy*

Indications: The key indication for this flower essence is a total preoccupation with self. These individuals are caught up with their own troubles, and are often hypochondriacs. They find it difficult to be alone, with an uncontrollable need to talk about themselves, and they are usually poor listeners. Unfortunately, they tend to alienate others, as friends and family often feel drained by the negative Heather's self-involvement. Most of us want relationships of mutual sharing—a two-way street, so to speak. Yet, Heather's sense of loneliness and great need for attention makes it hard to be able to give as well as receive. They're much too needy to consider others most of the time. This flower essence releases the extreme self-involvement of this state and brings awareness of being supportive to others—caring about others' needs and not just their own.

Examples: We can again look to the *Cheers* character, Cliff—himself this time—for an example of the Heather Type, in his constant self-absorption.

15–HOLLY

Botanical Name—*Ilex Aquifolium*
Vibration—*divine love*

Indications: The negative Holly state is portrayed by extreme feelings of hatred, suspicion, envy, jealously, and revenge. Holly assists us to open to a deep inner love that all possess within, as it releases these negative states of mind. This flower essence aids in releasing very negative and poisonous emotions, as it frees our true loving nature, making forgiveness possible. In many instances of divorce, which can bring up deep feelings of rage and hatred, Holly can assist in release and eventual forgiveness. Feelings of paranoia can also be treated with this flower essence.

There is an important point that needs to be addressed here, before continuing with the remaining flower essences. You do not choose Holly if you feel you want to be more loving—*unless* you are dealing with the aforementioned negative emotional states of the Holly profile. You do not take any flower essence to receive the positive quality it holds. You choose a particular flower essence only if you are experiencing the negative state that the flower essence addresses. Holly can open your natural loving nature, but only if you relate to the indications of the negative Holly state. This is true for all the flower essences, and important to remember in your selection process.

Examples: Again we turn to Ebenezer Scrooge, the main character portrayed in Charles Dickens' *A Christmas Carol*. This time it is Holly's profile that is revealed so well in the Scrooge we first meet as the story unfolds. He's depicted as cold-hearted, suspicious, and unable to care for anyone but himself. Another illustration is that of the character, J.R. Ewing, from the TV series, *Dallas*. He was also unloving, suspicious, envious, jealous, vengeful.

Terrorists, assassins, and recently, the unabomber, are other examples of the out of balance Holly state—to the extreme, as was the biblical character, Cain, the brother of Abel—all committing deplorable acts of cruelty and violence.

16–HONEYSUCKLE

Botanical Name—*Lonicera Caprifolium*
Vibration—*capacity for change*

Indications: This is the flower essence for those who seem lost in the past, longing for the good old days. The sense of nostalgia experienced prevents these individuals from living in the present in a productive and meaningful way. Many older people find themselves in this state, especially as partners and friends pass away. There doesn't seem to be much to live for anymore. Honeysuckle releases dwelling on past memories, and brings a new lease on life. It enables one to go out and meet new friends and develop new interests. Life becomes meaningful and vital again.

Holding onto the past is not just an issue with the elderly. It can arise at any age, depending on life circumstances. Many times, with divorce, it may be difficult not to think of the past and what was, preventing one from moving on in life. This flower essence is also excellent for young children who experience separation anxiety, as well as homesickness, making it difficult in going off to school, sleeping at a friend's, going away to camp, and other related situations of separation.

Examples: Dorothy, from *The Wizard of Oz*, is a wonderful illustration of this state. I can still see her clicking her little red shoes together and repeating, "There's no place like home, there's no place like home!" The character, Blanche DuBois, from Tennessee Williams's *A Streetcar Named Desire*, is another outstanding illustration of the Honeysuckle Type—lost in nostalgia for her lost youth and barely able to function in the present. Charles Dickens's book, *Great Expectations*, provides another superb example of this state. In this story, a character by the name of Mrs. Haversham, who was jilted just before her wedding day many years ago, continues to wear her wedding gown, which is now in tatters, seemingly living in her memories of what was to be. It would appear she certainly has refused to get on with her life!

17–HORNBEAM

Botanical Name—*Carpinus Betula*
Vibration—*inner vitality*

Indications: This is the flower essence for that Monday morning feeling—where you feel that your get-up-and-go has gotten up and gone. In this state you find that once you get started, you're fine. It's just that initial effort that seems so hard. There seems to be a weariness on some level. Your energy is a bit sapped. Many times, it is more on a mental level than physical one, and boredom may be at the root. Hornbeam assists those who feel a need for revitalization, and also helps with procrastination. This flower essence is also recommended for those who feel they may not be strong enough physically, with the need to strengthen the body, to build up their muscles.

Examples: The body builder types, such as Arnold Schwarzenegger, would exemplify this state, as does the Biblical character, Samson, who experienced a loss of vitality after having his hair cut off by Delilah!

18–IMPATIENS

Botanical Name—*Impatiens Gladulifera*
Vibration—*patience*

Indications: To get right at the heart of the matter *quickly*—Impatiens is for impatience! This personality type is a very independent, assertive, action-oriented individual who finds it difficult to work with others who are slower, and is intolerable of others who don't have the same energy drive, speed, and quickness of movement and perception. For this Type, "I want it done yesterday" isn't even soon enough! These individuals are easily irritated and restless, and don't take time to smell the flowers, coffee, or pizza!

Examples: New York City taxi drivers exemplify this negative state, par excellence. The White Rabbit, from Lewis Carroll's *Alice in Wonderland*, really gives you the sense of the impatient nature that this flower essence addresses! And with the dragging on of the O. J. Simpson trial, is there any question as to the sense of impatience that the jurors must have felt?

19–LARCH

Botanical Name—*Larix Decidua*
Vibration—*self-confidence*

Indications: The indications for this flower essence are low self-esteem and lack of self-confidence. Feelings of inferiority run deep in this Type. These individuals feel that success can never be theirs, and many times, don't even make the effort. As they anticipate failure in the end, theirs is an attitude of "why even bother." Larch puts us in touch with our own specialness. It brings awareness that we each have our own gift to share. This is another excellent flower essence for children with learning disabilities, as many have very little self-worth.

Examples: The roles played by Woody Allen in many of his movies illustrate this profile—all are characters who exhibit very little self-esteem and suffer from inferiority complexes.

20–MIMULUS

Botanical Name—*Mimulus Guttatus*
Vibration—*courage*

Indications: The indications for this flower essence are fears of *known* things—those you can name and put your finger on—such as fear of illness, fear of death, fear of not being financially secure, fear of loneliness, fear of intimacy, fear of public speaking, fear of animals, to mention a few of many possible fears. Phobias have also been successfully treated with Mimulus. This is the flower essence chosen for those who are extremely shy and timid individuals—characteristics which in most cases stem from a fear of being judged and rejected by others.

Examples: Little Miss Muffet, the nursery rhyme character who was frightened away by the spider who sat down beside her, is an example of the Mimulus state. Clark Kent, the alter-ego of Superman, portrays perfectly the profile of the Mimulus state. His persona is one of a timid and fearful man, seemingly lacking any courage. The Cowardly Lion from *The Wizard of Oz* is another illustration of the Mimulus state.

21–MUSTARD

Botanical Name—*Sinapis Arvensis*
Vibration—*cheerfulness*

Indications: This flower essence addresses another form of depression—one that comes upon us unexpectedly, and for no apparent reason, and then just as suddenly disappears. Mustard is for depression from an unknown, unconscious source, bringing feelings of doom and gloom. For those individuals who experience this state, Mustard eventually will bring to consciousness what it is that is causing the depression. This flower essence is excellent in cases of the "Postpartum Blues" which affects many new mothers.

Examples: The writings of Edgar Allan Poe, with gloom and doom soaking the pages, exemplify the negative Mustard state without peer!

22–OAK

Botanical Name—*Quercus Robur*
Vibration—*endurance*

Indications: This profile reflects very strong, capable, and self-reliant individuals who rarely seek help from others, possessing enormous endurance. However, sometimes they are too strong for their own good. They find it difficult to let go, ask for support, or take a break. Many of these individuals fall under the heading of workaholic—refusing to take time to rest, or heaven forbid, to play once in awhile!

In the extreme, even when ill, the Oak goes to work, ignoring the body's need for rest. The out of balance Oaks are very hard on themselves—with nose to the grindstone at all times. Being so dedicated and determined are admirable traits. Yet, if abusing the body and not considering its needs are continued, there eventually will be a price to pay.

There is another important point to mention before going further. The flower essences do not change the basic personality type. Their effect is to bring balance to the negative state. An Oak will always be an Oak, but now in equilibrium—no longer pushing beyond endurance, as before. This holds true for all the flower essences.

Examples: Abraham Lincoln was a genuine Oak. Reading about the hardships he encountered on the road to the Presidency, one is amazed at this man's strength and endurance in the face of all the obstacles he surmounted. *Star Trek's* Captain Kirk, is another depiction of the Oak Type—married to his ship the Enterprise, nothing could stand in the way of his dedication to her and his crew. He was responsible and hardworking to a fault in his role as captain and willing and able to withstand whatever challenges came his way. Mel Gibson's portrayal in the movie *Braveheart* is another quite profound example of this flower essence Type, as is Gloria Estefan, the pop singer whose back was broken and against all odds, has made a comeback. The biblical character Job as well, is another illustration of the Oak Type, as he persevered in the face of all obstacles.

23–OLIVE

Botanical Name—*Olea Europaea*
Vibration—*regeneration*

Indications: The indication for this flower essence is that of extreme exhaustion going far beyond the Hornbeam state. Here we have a situation where the physical system is totally depleted of energy, as during any major life-threatening illness, such as with cancer and AIDS, or after an operation, or even after childbirth. Olive is also of great help during emotional traumas, where the sense of loss is so extensive, one's physical energy has been depleted. It is suggested for any situation where major recovery and recuperation is indicated either emotionally or physically.

Examples: Greta Garbo's portrayal of *Camille*, in the movie of the same name, illustrates the Olive state, as she languishes from a terminal illness, her vitality all but depleted.

24–PINE

Botanical Name—*Pinus Sylvestris*
Vibration—*forgiveness*

Indications: The profile for this flower essence is that of the perfectionist. Nothing is ever good enough for the Pine, who feels there's always room for improvement. This perfectionism is only directed at themselves, however, and not expected of others. Self-criticism is the issue here. While beginning my studies of the Bach Flowers, my teacher remarked that Pine Types probably grew up with Beech parents who were intolerant of anything less than perfection. If their child brought home a 99 on a test, why wasn't it a 100? We can see, from this scenario, the potential for psychological damage. If children are constantly criticized in the formative years, they will most likely develop the feeling that nothing they do is really approved of.

Personal satisfaction is something hard for the Pine to relate to. Coupled often with this striving for perfection are feelings of guilt for not doing better. Many times, with the Pine profile, these individuals may blame themselves for others' mistakes. They are extremely apologetic. Out of balance Pines put much pressure on themselves with their demand for perfection at all times, setting high standards, yet feeling they can never attain them. By taking Pine, things are put into perspective. The Pine Types begin to realize they have done their best, and the pressure of feeling their efforts have not been good enough is released. Remember, the flower essences do not change the personality—selecting Pine doesn't change the desire for perfection, an intrinsic part of the Pine individual's personality, but brings balance to the pressure of the negative state.

Examples: The character Diane, portrayed by Shelley Long in the TV show *Cheers*, is the perfect example of the Pine Type. This character is unremittingly hard on herself, never feeling satisfied with her accomplishments—the perfectionist.

25–RED CHESTNUT

Botanical Name—*Aesculus Carnea*
Vibration—*solicitude*

Indications: The indications for this flower essence are major anxiety and overconcern for loved ones. Fears for the welfare of others are haunting and pervasive, bringing much stress in dealing with these constant worries. And constant is key here, as many of us worry from time to time about those we care for. But the Red Chestnut state is one of extreme fear—being overwrought and wrapped up in these stressful feelings continually—such as the mother, fearing for her child's safety constantly, or a wife, waiting for her husband to return from work. He's a half hour late. She finds herself imagining the worst. He must have had a car accident, and is now lying on the road critically wounded!

Examples: TV sitcom *All in the Family's* Edith Bunker again is used as a wonderful illustration, this time for the Red Chestnut state, as Edith is portrayed as constantly overwrought with concern for her family.

26–ROCK ROSE

Botanical Name—*Helianthemum Nummularium*
Vibration—*steadfastness*

Indications: Dr. Bach saw Rock Rose as the flower essence for emergency situations. It assists in releasing absolute terror and panic that usually emerges in any crisis. This flower essence is also excellent in calming the aftershocks of nightmares. The Rock Rose state is usually brief, and often related to a particular situation of extremity.

Examples: The character Ichabod Crane, from Washington Irving's *The Legend of Sleepy Hollow*, experienced and exemplified the Rock Rose state to the extreme while attempting to escape from the terrorizing specter of the headless horseman!

27–ROCK WATER

Vibration—*adaptability*

(There is no botanical name for 27 since it is the only remedy that is not a plant.)

Indications: This is the only Bach Essence not made from a plant or tree. It comes from healing waters where Dr. Bach worked and lived which he found to have special healing properties. Rock Water Types are those individuals who are self-denying, sometimes to the point of martyrdom. They have high ideals, and tend to be rigid in their disciplines. When out of balance, Rock Water Types can be too rigid and hard on themselves, slowly but surely squeezing the joy from their lives. The Rock Water sets an example for others, not by proselytizing, but by living and being the example. There is a strict adherence to a living style, or a personal, religious, or social discipline. The positive Rock Water deserves admiration. However, when out of balance, their personality traits can be potentially harmful to them. This flower essence brings balance to the overly rigid ideals of the Rock Water, instilling a sense of gentleness towards themselves.

Examples: Mahatma Gandhi personifies the Rock Water state in balance so perfectly. He had high ideals and followed a particular path in life, holding strongly to his convictions and beliefs. Several other examples of the Rock Water state are: Joan of Arc, Saint Francis, and Mother Teresa.

28–SCLERANTHUS

Botanical Name—*Scleranthus Annuus*
Vibration—*balance*

Indications: "Do I buy a Chevy or a Toyota? Do I choose teal or silver? Do I want a 2-door or 4-door?" Decisions, decisions, decisions! When faced with choosing between two things, and we find we cannot make up our minds, then it's time to turn to Scleranthus. People of this Type are very indecisive in their lives—vacillating back and forth in making their choices—they waffle. This flower essence is also helpful for those who have a tendency towards mood swings, experiencing extremes of joy/sadness, optimism/pessimism, etc. Scleranthus is the flower essence for balance on many levels, and also extremely helpful for motion sickness.

Examples: Because President Clinton seems so indecisive, he might be helped by Scleranthus. Shakespeare's *Hamlet* also exhibited the Scleranthus state in his "To Be or Not To Be" soliloquy.

29–STAR OF BETHLEHEM

Botanical Name—*Ornitholagum Umbellatum*
Vibration—*restoration*

Indications: The indications for this very special flower essence are deep feelings of grief due to the loss of a loved one, either through death or separation of any kind, as well as any physical or emotional trauma we've experienced. The trauma may have occurred many years ago, or yesterday—any trauma, including physical or emotional abuse, an accident, or trauma from an operation. It seems that the body holds on to shock and trauma long after the fact. Many times, even years later, delayed effects may manifest as physical symptoms, nervous breakdowns, anxiety attacks, depression, etc. For many, true healing can only begin after the release of any trauma. The vibration of this flower essence works at the cellular level and releases any traumatic experience from the cellular memory itself. Star of Bethlehem is highly recommended for survivors of incest, physical/sexual abuse, rape, and those suffering from post traumatic stress disorder. Both mothers and infants can also be helped in releasing the trauma of the birth process.

Examples: *Gone With the Wind's* Scarlett O'Hara was in a Star of Bethlehem state after losing her beloved home Tara, as was Olympic figure skater Nancy Kerrigan after her physical assault.

30–SWEET CHESTNUT

Botanical Name—*Castanea Sativa*
Vibration—*release*

Indications: This is another flower essence that treats depression—a depression that is more profound than that of the Gentian or Gorse states. In the Sweet Chestnut state, one feels as though plunged into a black hole filled with darkness and despair, unable to go on. Yet, so weakened by despondency, there is no energy left to end it all. This state is probably the most severe depression that can be experienced. It leaves a sense of isolation so great that even God seems out of reach. Sweet Chestnut brings solace when the limits of our endurance have been tapped.

Examples: Shakespeare's *Hamlet* is again used to now illustrate the profile of Sweet Chestnut. The angst that Hamlet experienced in his soul searching soliloquy, "To Be or Not To Be," gives us a sense of the depths of his emotional pain.

31–VERVAIN

Botanical Name—*Verbena Officinalis*
Vibration—*restraint*

Indications: Those people who are strong-willed individuals, always having to be right, and also needing to convince others of their stand fit this profile. They will argue to the death defending their beliefs and opinions! This is the personality Type of the teacher, the prophet, or the proselytizer. There is high personal energy in Vervain individuals, and a tendency to be a bit on the hyper side at times, making them predisposed to burn-out. When out of balance, the need to sell their opinions to others becomes a problem. They force their beliefs on all those they encounter, thus alienating themselves. Vervain Types in balance are special teachers who stimulate and inspire those whose lives they touch—without using that 2 by 4! They live their truths and are a model for others.

Examples: Dr. Martin Luther King beautifully exemplifies the balanced Vervain Type in his "I have a dream" speech. President John F. Kennedy also typifies the positive Vervain Type in his moving address to the country, as he admonished us to "Ask not what your country can do for you, but what you can do for your country." We can also recognize the Vervain profile in former First Lady Eleanor Roosevelt, a great humanitarian; actress Jane Fonda, with her stand on the Vietnam War some years ago; evangelist Billy Graham, and lawyer Johnnie Cochran, in his defense of O. J. Simpson. Talk show hostess Oprah Winfrey is another inspiring example of Vervain, as well as the fictitious character Robin Hood, who robbed from the rich to give to the poor as he lived by his beliefs.

32–VINE

Botanical Name—*Vitis Vinifera*
Vibration—*right use of authority*

Indications: "I am in the position of authority and control here. We do it *my* way and there is no room for discussion." This dictatorial statement could have easily been made by a Vine out of balance. This personality Type is domineering, controlling, and inflexible. They believe *their* way is the only way, and brook no interference. On the positive side, when in balance, Vines are born leaders, organized, in control of themselves, and very together. They are capable individuals who take charge and get things done. Many look to the Vine for leadership and direction. Rigidity is not healthy, nor is shouldering the entire responsibility, as Vines tend to do. This flower essence brings flexibility and the willingness to listen to others, and creates a beneficent leader who is appreciated, respected, and looked up to, rather than avoided, feared, and disliked.

Examples: When the Vine is out of balance, we have the dictator—a Napoleon, a Hitler, a Saddam Hussein, who all exemplify the negative Vine profile. Called Chairman of the Board by his friends, Frank Sinatra appears to have the qualities of a Vine. The popular ballad "My Way," which was written especially for him by Paul Anka, captures the very essence of Mr. Sinatra and his life, and is an amazing portrayal of the Vine Type. My sense is that Elvis Presley, forever immortalized as the King by his adoring fans, was a Vine personality, as well as having exhibited traits of the Agrimony, Crab Apple, and Pine Types. Many biographies have been written, portraying Elvis as a man who held a tight rein over his entourage, was addicted to drugs and alcohol, was overly concerned about his appearance and subsequent weight gain, and was a perfectionist in his work.

33—WALNUT

Botanical Name—*Juglans Regia*
Vibration—*unaffectedness*

Indications: There are many uses for this remarkable flower essence. It is one of the most often selected of all 38, and for good reason. Walnut's indications are for all transitional periods in life—teething, puberty, beginning a career, marriage, becoming a parent, the empty nest syndrome, divorce, retirement, and menopause, to give several illustrations of major life changes. Walnut is for any time or period in life that requires adjustment to new situations. It brings to us an ease and more confidence to move through these transitions smoothly and with less stress. It assists us to more easily break the links or ties with the past that may bind us to the old ways—as in a relationship that isn't working out, yet we fear making the break and going it alone.

Walnut is known as the "Link Breaker," and is another flower essence that assists in releasing drug dependency. It also enables individuals to steer their own ships, and not be influenced by others who disagree with a course they have chosen (as with the dominating Vine Type father, or possessive Chicory Type mother who may do their best to control or manipulate their adult children's path in life according to their personal agenda). Walnut assists in remaining true to convictions and in being master of one's own life. It helps individuals to not be swayed by what others think is best for them. Perhaps the course of history would have been changed if Walnut had been available to Adam and Eve!

This flower essence is a protection against all outside influences, and has been used successfully in treating allergies for this reason. It is also a wonderful support for all those who work in the healing field—counselors, body workers, nurses, etc., as it also protects against any client's potentially draining energy.

Examples: Dr. Bach was a strong Walnut Type. He cared so little for what the medical establishment thought of him that he jeopardized his medical career to remain true to his calling. The singer and actress Madonna is another marvelous illustration of the Walnut Type. She certainly appears to be unaffected by the influence of others, and has been charting her own unique, if sometimes outrageous, course in life.

34–WATER VIOLET

Botanical Name—*Hottonia Palustris*
Vibration—*humility*

Indications: Water Violet individuals are proud, aloof, independent people who go through life doing their work quietly, preferring to be left alone. They are gentle souls who do their own thing—not easily influenced by others, nor do they have the need to influence others. The problem with the out of balance Water Violet is their tendency towards isolation. No person is an island. We are all connected on some level, and need human contact for our growth. Those who relate to the Water Violet profile, as well as to Oak and Rock Water, may feel there is no need for change. These three personality Types have many worthy qualities. This is true so long as balance is maintained. Stress to the system begins once balance is lost. Water Violet finds it uncomfortable relating with others. There is a tendency to become loners and shun contact which prevents them from truly knowing themselves. In addition to this pervading quality of detachment, the Water Violet profile may have feelings of superiority involved—which is actually well-founded. Water Violet is a special teacher and leader. Others look to them for their sense of calmness and self-assurance. They have gifts to share with humanity.

Examples: The TV and movie character, Mr. Spock, of *Star Trek* fame, shows many of the Water Violet tendencies especially with his detached demeanor. Jackie Kennedy with her strong sense of pride, represents another Water Violet profile, as does actor James Dean, known by his peers as a loner. The actress Greta Garbo is remembered by many not only for her great dramatic talent, but for her extreme sense of privacy. In her inimitable accent, she reportedly spoke the following words, "I vant to be alawn," words that will always be a testament to her personality. And these are the very words that are at the heart of the Water Violet profile.

35–WHITE CHESTNUT

Botanical Name—*Aesculus Hippocastanum*
Vibration—*tranquillity*

Indications: The White Chestnut state is expressed during those times when the mind seems to race on and on, or it feels like a record has gotten stuck in the groove—repeating the same obsessive thought many times over. Peace of mind is nowhere to be found in this state. We find ourselves plagued by unwanted thoughts, and can't seem to focus or concentrate on anything else.

In this state as well, sleeping patterns may be disrupted. We are unable to shut off the mind when going to sleep, or may wake up in the middle of the night as the mind continues to work overtime. Sometimes we wake well before it's time to start the day and are unable to go back to sleep. White Chestnut assists in releasing these persistent, unwanted, and sometimes obsessive thought patterns, as it brings a stillness and peace to the mind. This flower essence is another often used for children with learning disabilities, as an aid in concentration.

Examples: Shakespeare's *Lady MacBeth* was suffering from the White Chestnut state, in her obsession with washing her hands to remove imagined blood stains, as she continually repeated, "Out, out, damned spot!"

36–WILD OAT

Botanical Name—*Bromus Ramosus*
Vibration—*purposefulness*

Indications: "What is the meaning and purpose of my life? What direction am I to go in?" For those with these questions, Wild Oat, known as the "Pathfinder," may be the catalyst in discovering the answers. Wild Oat's profile includes dissatisfaction, boredom, and feeling unfulfilled in our present work. There's a futile kind of feeling that doesn't go away as we continue on the same road. It's true that we all need to support ourselves, yet, hopefully, we can also find what it is we love to do. Wild Oat assists us in handling and dealing with present circumstances by releasing the attached stress and restlessness. It helps us find contentment in what we're doing or, if necessary, opens us to the courage needed to leave so we may go out and find what our calling is.

Examples: The character Walter Mitty exemplifies the Wild Oat state, with his constant changing of occupations and search for his path.

37–WILD ROSE

Botanical Name—*Rosa Canina*
Vibration—*inner motivation*

Indications: The profile of this flower essence is that of apathy and resignation. These Types feel that their lot in life can never change, and have totally accepted their circumstances as irreversible. The Wild Rose individual feels as though there is no hope left to live a richer life. There isn't even depression anymore—just a pervasive numbness, as though the spark of life has just about gone out. Many who suffer from life-threatening disease are prone to this state, as well as invalids and the handicapped, and those who see themselves as victims of abuse. This flower essence brings the realization that there are choices, and it's not too late to have a more meaningful life.

Examples: Willy Loman, in Arthur Miller's *Death of a Salesman*, exemplifies the apathy and resignation of the Wild Rose state. The baby duckling in Hans Christian Andersen's story, who faces almost insurmountable rejection, also exemplifies the Wild Rose state.

38–WILLOW

Botanical Name—*Salix Vitellina*
Vibration—*personal responsibility*

Indications: The last but definitely not the least of the 38 individual Bach Flower Essences is Willow. The indications for this flower essence are bitterness and resentment. Willow individuals feel that life has given them a raw deal—whether it be their mother or father they blame, or the universe itself.

They see themselves as victims. Willow personalities take no responsibility for their lives, blaming others, or circumstances and events, for the causes of their misery. We all need to realize that on some level, we—not others—are responsible for the place we are in. At age thirty-five or forty, we need to stop blaming our parents for any hurts or actions that took place thirty years ago or perhaps, what they didn't do for us. It's time to grow up and get a life! At some point we need to finally release the blame we hold. We're only hurting ourselves with the toxins produced in our bodies by these negative emotions. We need to forgive and let go of the past. We also need to understand, although it may be difficult to see, that our parents or anyone else we may hold grievances against have been doing the best they are capable of, even if we perceive it has been hurtful. This is not to excuse wrongful behavior. Yet eventually, for our own peace of mind and state of our health itself, we need to move past what was. Willow assists in releasing bitterness and resentment. It brings awareness of our responsibility for our own life, and helps us to see that all we experience are lessons and opportunities for our personal growth—even when we may not be given any reasons as to why we need to go through these lessons.

Examples: Tonya Harding, Olympic figure skater, appears to experienced the Willow state in her resentment of her rival, Nancy Kerrigan, as well as the Holly state by her subsequent attack on Nancy.

Regrettably, a deeply poignant illustration of the Willow state, as well as Holly and Star of Bethlehem states, has recently been televised nationally. With the tragic murders of Nicole Simpson and Ron Goldman, many of us have been witness to their families' extreme emotional turmoil and loss—clearly depicting the indications for the Bach Flower Essences Willow, Holly, and Star of Bethlehem.

We have now completed the Indications for each of the 38 individual Bach Flowers. If you wish to obtain a deeper understanding of Dr. Bach's insights into healing, as well as the indications for each of the 38 flower essences in his own words, I highly recommend reading *The Bach Flower Essences*, as well as *The Original Writings of Edward Bach*. Please refer to the section on Recommended Reading for further information.

One final Bach Flower preparation—Rescue Remedy—remains to be addressed. As there is so much to share regarding this extraordinary combination formula, the next chapter is devoted to an in depth exploration of Rescue.

"Thus we see that our conquest of disease will mainly depend upon the following: the realization of the Divinity within our nature and our consequent power to overcome all that is wrong; secondly, the knowledge that the basic cause of disease is due to disharmony between the personality and the Soul; and thirdly, our willingness and ability to discover the fault which is causing such a conflict; and fourthly, the removal of any such fault by developing the opposing virtue."

Dr. Edward Bach
Heal Thyself

Rescue Remedy: Dr. Bach's "Emergency" Formula

In addition to the 38 individual flower essences that Dr. Bach developed, there is also one special combination of his flower essences that was created specifically for Emergency Stress Relief, known as Rescue Remedy. This outstanding preparation is composed of five of the original 38 flower essences, and can be used with great success in any emergency situation. The five flower essences comprising Rescue Remedy are Clematis, addressing dizziness or loss of consciousness; Cherry Plum, addressing loss of mental and/or physical control; Impatiens, addressing emotional tension and/or pain; Rock Rose, addressing panic and terror; and Star of Bethlehem, addressing emotional or physical trauma and/or grief and loss.

Rescue Remedy is highly effective and always brings instant relief in cases of extreme stress when a person is close to the edge. This is the only Bach Flower Essence that has an *immediate* Reaction Time, with its effects felt usually within 15 to 20 minutes. It may also be taken as often as needed without fear of overdosing, as all the flower essences are totally safe and gentle, natural and non-toxic preparations.

Any crisis condition warrants its use. To illustrate, some of the many possible crisis situations that Rescue Remedy eases are: anxiety attacks, grief, shock and trauma, panic and hysteria. Even minor incidents that cause stress and anxiety, such as arguments, exams, public speaking, job interviews, visits to the doctor or dentist—all are addressed and feelings calmed with Rescue Remedy. Once you've personally experienced its amazing effectiveness, you'll want to keep Rescue Remedy available for any emergency situation that should unexpectedly arise. Rescue Remedy also comes in a cream formula, with the addition of Crab Apple, the flower essence for cleansing. It is used for burns, cuts, rashes, insect bites and stings, bruises, and even helps with blemishes. It is also wonderfully soothing for tired eyes, as well as easing nipple soreness that many mothers who breast feed sometimes experience.

Several actual experiences with Rescue Remedy taken from my client files are now presented as illustrations of its remarkable efficacy.

Case Histories:

Kim woke in the middle of the night, finding herself extremely nauseous. As she rushed to the bathroom feeling she might vomit, she also experienced dizziness. She had been using the Bach Flowers for some time, and always kept a bottle of Rescue Remedy in the medicine chest. She immediately reached for it and sank down to the floor, feeling faint. She managed to put several drops in her mouth, and within minutes, the dizziness passed. Although still nauseous, she was unable to throw up. She put four to five drops of Rescue Remedy into a half glass of water and brought it back to bed with her. She sipped every few minutes, and within fifteen to twenty minutes her nausea abated enough for her to be able to go back to sleep. When she awoke the next morning, her experience of the previous evening seemed like a bad dream. She later called me to share her delight at how helpful Rescue had been.

Sue was experiencing a major anxiety attack when she called me. She was restless and pacing, feeling overwhelmingly agitated and unable to calm herself. I suggested she put several drops of Rescue Remedy into a half glass of water and sip every five minutes. I asked her to call me back in a half hour. When she called back, she was amazed at how calm and relaxed she now was. Whatever she had been experiencing was totally gone. She told me how glad she was that she had taken my advice in our last consultation, when I recommended she have Rescue Remedy on hand for unexpected crises.

Ann recently reported this incident to me—one concerning her mother. They bowled together, and one day her mom began to feel dizzy. Ann is "hooked on Bach," and always carries Rescue Remedy in her purse just in case. Well, it really came in handy in this situation. Ann gave her mother some Rescue Remedy in half a glass of water, advising her to sip every five minutes. She did as instructed, and within about fifteen minutes or so, her mom was feeling up to resuming her bowling. Her dizziness was completely gone! Ann's mother now carries her own bottle of Rescue Remedy in her purse.

When Jim came for a recent Bach consultation, he mentioned that his dog, Hercules, was afraid of thunderstorms. He wondered if the flower essences could also help his pet. I suggested he administer some Rescue Remedy the next time it stormed. An opportunity soon arose, and Jim called to let me know that Hercules now lives up to his name!

Vicki had recently lost her father. She had been in deep emotional pain over her loss for several weeks when a friend and client of mine told her about the Bach Flowers. Vicki came to see me and soon was using Rescue Remedy, at first taking it as often as she felt the need, then eventually four times a day. Within the week, she reported that her grieving had eased up considerably and she was much more comfortable. Where she was finding it hard to cope with everyday life before, caused by her depression over her dad's death, she was now able to resume her normal routine.

Tom, my brother-in-law, had come to visit several summers ago. I couldn't help but notice his swollen hand. I had never seen anything like this before—it was three times its normal size! When I asked what had happened, he said he had been stung by a bee earlier in the day. I told him I had something I felt could help his discomfort, and asked if he'd allow me to put some Rescue Remedy cream on his hand. He agreed and within the hour, the swelling had been markedly reduced. We put on a second application and by the time he left, his hand was almost back to normal. He was amazed with the results and asked me to order some for him. I have to honestly admit that I was almost as amazed, as was Tom, by the dramatic change.

Lyn, after a recent consultation, learned to always keep Rescue liquid and cream on hand. She recently called to let me know how helpful they had been after badly burning her arm and how glad she was that she remembered to use them. She first made a compress with the liquid, and held it on her arm for about one half hour. Initially, the throbbing pain was unbearable, but soon after applying the compress, the pain quickly subsided. She then applied some cream on the effected area and bandaged it. The next morning she discovered how beautifully it had healed. A water blister had developed, which she broke. Once again she applied the cream, and again bandaged her wound. All pain had disappeared and by the next day, it was well on its way to total healing.

Esther, a new friend with whom I had shared my work with the Bach Flowers, had recently gotten some Rescue cream not knowing how soon she'd need it. One morning, just as her eight-year-old son Adam was leaving for school, he fell against the storm door, badly banging his forehead. He sustained a large bruise which was beginning to swell. Esther immediately reached for the Rescue cream and generously applied it to Adam's wound. After waiting a bit to determine if her son was OK, and not in need of further medical attention, she sent him off to school. He agreed to take the Rescue cream with him and apply it several more times. Esther reported that she was amazed when she later saw her son. She could find no evidence of the bruise or any swelling that had earlier appeared. She remarked to me, "It seemed like a miracle!"

Mary, another Bach Practitioner, shared this experience with me. Her elderly mother had fallen and bruised her shoulder. She called Mary for advice as it was bruised. Mary told her to apply Rescue cream to the area which she did, as well as place a bandage on it. The next day, Mary came by to check on her mother. It seems her mom had only applied the Rescue cream to a portion of the bruise where she had bandaged it. When Mary removed the bandage, the skin here was completely free of discoloration.

However, the surrounding area that hadn't been treated was still black and blue!

Marc, my son, had badly cut his finger late one evening. It really needed a few stitches, but as it was after 11 P.M., we decided to treat the wound with Rescue. We first made a compress with the liquid. Once the bleeding stopped, we applied the cream and bandaged it. The next morning we again applied the cream with a fresh bandage. Within three days the cut had completely healed with no evidence of it ever being there. The cut had been pretty deep. It was remarkable that it had healed so quickly, and without any scarring.

I could go on and on in sharing the remarkable effects of Rescue Remedy liquid and cream. The above experiences should suffice in giving you a pretty good picture of the many situations that Rescue assists with. If you try no other flower essence, I deeply urge you to at least experience Rescue Remedy. It is my opinion that no medicine chest should be without it. Carry Rescue in your purse and glove compartment of your car for any unexpected emergency situation that arises.

Bach Flower Preparation and Use

You should now have a firm handle on those essences which relate to your emotional issues and negative states of mind, and are ready to experience for yourself the remarkable efficacy of this very special self-help system.

Once you have your flower essences on hand, there are many different ways to use them. You may take your drops directly from the concentrate bottles. However, I would like to recommend an easier and more economical way of taking them, especially when taking several flower essences at once. You can combine your flower essences together in a Personal Dilution Bottle.

As the flower essences are homeopathic in nature, it is possible to dilute them one time without changing their strength. For some, this concept may be difficult to accept, and bring concern that the potency is weakened by diluting. Let me reassure you that this is not the case with the Bach Flower Essences. Know that they may be safely diluted according to directions that now follow without disturbing their original potency.

You will need a one-ounce amber dropper bottle into which you place two or three drops of each flower essence selected. The *only* exception is Rescue Remedy. Because it is a combination formula, you will need to use four to five drops of Rescue. Remember—it is suggested that no more than *seven* flower essences are to be used at any one time. Rescue is considered *one* flower essence when combining it in your dilution bottle. If you are in need of more than two or three of the flower essences in Rescue, it may be helpful to use Rescue itself, rather than the individual ones, to keep the number of flower essences from exceeding seven.

Sterilize the bottle before you prepare it with your personal formula. Boil both the glass bottle and rubber dropper top for at least fifteen minutes. It is perfectly safe to boil the rubber top, and it will not be harmed by boiling. It is not necessary to re-sterilize your bottle after the initial preparation, so long as you continue to use the same flower essences. When your bottle is empty, simply add the water, flower essences, and preservative as before. However, when you find the need to change any of the flower essences you have been using, it then becomes necessary to again sterilize your bottle to ensure the removal of the vibration of previous flower essences.

After placing your flower essences into your bottle, add a teaspoon of *one* of the following as a preservative: either apple cider vinegar, brandy, or vegetable glycerin may be used. As the flower essences are not to be refrigerated, but simply kept in a cool, dark place, they need a preservative to prevent spoilage. Now, fill the rest of your bottle with spring water and shake well. You are ready to begin your flower essence use.

The dosage is at least *four* drops from your dilution bottle under the tongue for a minimum of *four* times daily. If you choose to take the flower essences directly from the concentrate bottle, you need to take *two* to *three* drops from each bottle that you are presently using. If you are using Rescue, it's *four* to *five* drops of the concentrate. You can see how much more convenient it is to take your drops from a single bottle with all your flower essences combined than it would be to do so from several different bottles. You may also place a few drops from the concentrate into a half glass of water. Each sip is considered a single dose. Again, I remind you, in most cases you probably won't feel the effect of the flower essences immediately, with the exception of Rescue Remedy. The other 38 individual flower essences usually need to be taken for a one to two month period, with your personal commitment to use them regularly before you may begin to feel their subtle effects. And reaction time does vary with each person.

In regard to limiting the number of flower essences to the general recommendation of seven, one of the most helpful and effective ways to do this is by using an Intensity Scale. This simple technique may be done by noting on a piece of paper the flower essences you wish to take. Review each one, determining how often you are experiencing their indications. Is this once a week, every few days, or every day? You will then need to rate all tentative selections. Give each a numerical value between one and ten, depending on how intense each issue is for you. Give the highest value to the most stressful.

To illustrate this process, perhaps you've related to ten flower essences, and Mimulus is among them—for the constant fears you feel. This issue is one you face daily. You would give Mimulus a "ten." Another of the ten flower essences you are considering may be Cerato—for your inability to make your own decisions. Yet, you notice that although you have a need to go to others for advice, sometimes you are able to make your own decisions without asking others' opinions. Cerato would be a "six" perhaps. You continue this procedure with all ten flower essences. Once you've rated each one, simply select those with the highest numbers. These represent your most intense issues. Hopefully, this process will have narrowed down your selections to the recommended maximum of seven. If you are unsuccessful on the first try, simply repeat this process until only seven remain.

One of the most common occurrences with Bach Flower usage is referred to as the "Peeling Effect." When you feel you are ready to stop taking your original selections—and this is something only you can determine—you'll probably discover, as have so many others, that different issues have now surfaced and are now also ready to be released. It seems that in our healing process, as one or more surface issues are resolved, other underlying and deeper issues may begin to emerge into consciousness. A helpful analogy is that of the onion with its many layers. As the top layer is peeled, the next layer is revealed, and then another, until the core is reached. The uncovering of deeper, unresolved emotional issues is a normal and continuing process in your personal growth throughout life. As this peeling effect occurs for you, simply repeat the selection process in choosing new flower essences that relate to the issue or issues now being revealed. Simply re-read the indications for each of the flower essences previously presented, for further assistance with your new selections.

For those who are alcohol sensitive and wondering if they can safely use the flower essences which contain a significant amount of alcohol in the concentrate form, the answer is absolutely yes. There are several ways to prepare and use the flower essences, dispelling the alcohol, if this is a question or concern for you. By putting the drops directly into hot water, the alcohol is totally evaporated. Making the dilution bottle as previously instructed is another way to reduce the alcohol content. Do not select brandy as your preservative. Also, the flower essences may be directly applied to the pulse points of the skin, itself. And one last possible application suggested for alcohol sensitivity—mist the flower essences into the air from a spray bottle. Any one of these alternate ways of using the flower essences has been found to be just as effective as taking them by mouth.

Another possible circumstance to be aware of, although very infrequently experienced when using the flower essences, is something called the "Healing Crisis." In any healing process, in some cases, it appears that a situation will get worse before it gets better. This takes place in traditional medical treatment, in counseling, in all healing modalities. A common illustration of this is a simple fever. We have all experienced how this condition seems to reach a certain point before it can break. In simplest terms, this is what is known as a healing crisis.

As the flower essences bring up our emotional issues for release, sometimes an individual may feel an issue growing more intense instead of easing, at the outset. If this happens to you, know that this experience is very short-lived, usually disappearing within one to two days at the most. The Bach Flowers themselves do not cause any side-effects. This healing crisis is but a part of the healing process itself. The following suggestions will help you to move past this situation. You may use Rescue, along with the other flower essences you are using, to ease what is taking place and push through the crisis. You may also decide to stop taking whichever flower essence you sense may be causing you this emotional discomfort. And know that this *is* an option—you may not be ready to deal with this particular issue at this time. And this is OK, as your healing process is very personal and not to be judged, even by you! Honor your feelings, and if you are too uncomfortable, discontinue use for awhile. You may also want to continue taking Rescue for a few days until you feel all discomfort has passed. Please be gentle with yourself. Don't force any healing. Go at your own pace. Know that you are in charge of your own healing process here. And again, I repeat—this healing crisis is *rarely* experienced.

Dr. Bach developed his flower essences not only for acute emergency situations, and for the healing of deep-seated emotional issues and negative states of mind but also for one's personality makeup, to prevent the manifestation of disease in the future. Therefore, it is helpful to know which of the flower essences relate to your *personality*. The flower essences that address the personality and long-standing feelings that may cause an individual to go out of balance are called "Type" flower essences. These have the ability to transform your character flaws or weaknesses into your greatest strengths.

Type flower essences are those that relate to our Basic Nature. Most of us usually have several, as we are diverse beings, and there is usually a combination of flower essences which represent our unique complexities. You probably recognized several of your own Type flower essences while going over the 38 Indications, ones that spoke to you, that you identified as parts of your personality characteristics. Our Type flower essences are ones we will never outgrow, and have the ability to open us to our most positive states of being.

By taking the flower essences that depict your personality, you are assisting your system's harmony and balance at all times. This is a key concept with Bach Flower usage. By taking your personality Type flower essences, even if the characteristics addressed by them are in balance for you, you are ensuring the continuation of this state. And this is an important concept in assisting you in your healing process. Take the time to discover your Type flower essences, and use them even when you feel balanced, as a preventative.

Dr. Bach felt that if individuals could determine their personality Type flower essences, these would then be the only ones needed, regardless of what was taking place in their lives, and the emotional responses to these situations. This is possible because the Type flower essences bring one's basic disposition into balance. Any ensuing conflict or disharmony, therefore, would also be balanced easily.

One last factor that needs to be addressed in regard to flower essence use is the question of "Integrity." Many have brought up the question of the feasibility of giving the flower essences to others without their knowledge or approval (more likely, to help themselves more than the person they'd like to give the flower essences to. Perhaps they are dealing with a Beech or Vine Type!) Although the flower essences are effective regardless of the awareness of an individual, this question is really one of ethical principles.

Without the intent to preach here, I personally do not believe we have the right to force change on another, or to take actions along these lines without another's approval, even if it may be for their own good. Just as Dr. Bach believed that no one has the right to interfere in our life, he also believed that we do not have the right to interfere in another's life. He stated in *Free Thyself*, "God gave us each our birthright, an individuality all our own...He gave us each our own particular path to follow...Let us see to it that not only do we allow no interference, but even more important, that we, in no way whatsoever, interfere with any other single human being." As we take our freedom to be ourselves, we need to give this same freedom to others. When we share the Bach Flowers with others, it must be with their awareness and approval. Although I have stated my feelings regarding this question, and also shared those of Dr. Bach, you are, of course, free to determine your own position with this issue.

However, there are several situations where receiving another's approval is not possible, as with an individual being unconscious, or mentally incompetent, as well as with young children under our care. They are all unable to help themselves. In situations such as these, with our positive intention of bringing relief to others we may be responsible for, there would be no breach of integrity in our use of the Bach Flowers. To administer the Bach Flowers to an unconscious individual, simply moisten the lips with several drops of the essence, apply to the pulse points, or mist the room with a spray bottle containing at least eight drops of each of the flower essences you wish to use.

Bach Flowers for Common Life Situations

The remaining chapters are devoted to bringing to you many of the diversified uses of the Bach Flowers, from various emotionally challenging "Life Situations" we all have in common to flower essence application with animals and even plants! Cases from my own practice will be presented as illustrations for you, to assist you in your own understanding and use of the Bach Flowers.

There are many difficult and stressful life situations that we all will face at one time or another as a part of the human condition. There is no way of avoiding them. A loved one dying, facing our own mortality, a painful divorce, the loss of a career, a diagnosis of cancer or other life-threatening diseases, are just a few of the many devastating emotional traumas we may experience. Although we cannot always prevent the course that our life may run, we do have help in dealing with the repercussions of emotional stresses we may encounter—with the Bach Flowers.

BEREAVEMENT

In times of deep grief and loss experienced with the death of a loved one, the flower essences most often indicated are Walnut for the state of transition; Star of Bethlehem for grief and loss, and possibly shock and trauma, if the death was sudden; Honeysuckle for nostalgia and living in past memories; Willow for resentment towards the one who died and/or the situation itself; and Sweet Chestnut for deep depression. Agrimony may also be indicated if there is denial and repression of feelings of grief. If the loss is emotionally devastating, bringing on physical exhaustion, there may also be a need for Olive. And Rescue Remedy itself (which also contains Star of Bethlehem) is extremely helpful.

DEATH AND DYING

In facing our own death and the issues that confront us, or in assisting another who is making this final transition, many of the same flower essences are indicated as for the loss of a loved one. It is sad that there is so much avoidance and fear surrounding the death experience. We do ourselves a terrible disservice in our culture. Many people find themselves isolated and alone in their final days, with friends and relatives tiptoeing around the truth, caught up in their own denial and fear. The following flower essences are generally suggested to bring comfort to the dying. Agrimony assists with denial and brings the ability to face our deepest feelings over death. Aspen eases the fear of the unknown. Either Gorse or Sweet Chestnut may be indicated for feelings of hopelessness or extreme anguish when confronted with death. There may be a need for Holly during the initial phase when anger and rage may surface. Mimulus brings courage and releases fear. Olive may be indicated where total exhaustion from infirmity is experienced. Red Chestnut is needed when there is overconcern for how loved ones will manage without them. Star of Bethlehem comforts feelings of grief and loss. Walnut is always indicated for this time of major transition. Wild Rose may sometimes be needed if apathy or resignation sets in. And Willow may be a consideration when feelings of bitterness or resentment develop.

DIVORCE

During and after a divorce the flower essences most often indicated, especially for those deeply hurt, are Star of Bethlehem for grief and loss; Mimulus for fear of being alone; Honeysuckle for living in the past; Walnut for breaking links with the past life, and the state of transition; Holly for rage and hatred towards the ex-spouse; and perhaps, Willow for bitterness and resentment; Larch for lack of self-confidence in making it alone; and, for possible depression, Sweet Chestnut or Gorse, depending on the severity of the depression. Olive may also be indicated for the total exhaustion possibly caused by this emotionally stressful situation. Pine is another consideration, when there are feelings of guilt and self-blame involved that are unwarranted.

LOSS OF CAREER

With the loss of a career, the flower essences most often indicated are Rescue Remedy for anxiety and panic; Mimulus for all known fears that may come up in this situation; Wild Oat for considering a new direction in life; Impatiens for impatience while going through this transition Walnut for the state of transition itself; Larch for lack of self-worth; either Holly or Willow for feelings of rage or bitterness; as well as Star of Bethlehem (which is also in Rescue Remedy) for grief and loss. Gorse may also be indicated for feelings of hopelessness.

LIFE-THREATENING ILLNESSES (AIDS, CANCER, HEART DISEASE, ETC.)

The flower essences most often indicated are Rescue Remedy for the terror and panic; Mimulus for fear of death; Gorse for hopelessness, or Sweet Chestnut for extreme anguish; Wild Rose for apathy and resignation; Olive for physical exhaustion; and Crab Apple, as a cleanser. Holly or Willow may also be indicated for feelings of rage or bitterness, as well as Agrimony for denial.

The above life-challenging scenarios just presented are examples of some of the many different emotional states that can come up during such experiences. Not everyone will experience them in the same way, nor need the same flower essences, nor are these states described definitive. These situations have been generalized so as to give you a deeper understanding of the various negative emotional states possible and the 38 flower essences, including Rescue Remedy that address them.

The illustrations that now follow are of clients I have counseled during similar life challenging situations. They are presented as more specific and individualized illustrations, to bring further clarity and understanding in your use and practice of the Bach Flowers.

Case Histories:

Barbara, a woman in her early sixties, had just lost her husband. His death triggered deep depression, with feelings of abandonment and fear. She withdrew into herself, unable to continue with daily life. Her daughter Joan became increasingly worried over her mother's emotional state and felt her mother needed help in overcoming her bereavement. Fortunately, Barbara agreed to seek help and an appointment was set up for a Bach Flower consultation. When I saw Barbara, her deep emotional pain was evident. Her face was pale with dark circles under her eyes. It was hard for her to talk without dissolving into tears. She expressed deep grief, as well as fear of being on her own now. Her husband had been her strength, she advised. She didn't know if she could manage on her own. She also expressed resentment at her husband dying and leaving her alone—"How could he do this to me?" she bitterly cried. (In my studies of death and dying, I have come to learn that it is not uncommon for those who experience the death of a loved one to feel deep resentment towards the one who died. It appears this is part of the grieving process itself—one of the stages that needs to be moved through).

After listening to Barbara share her feelings over her situation, I suggested the following flower essences which related to the negative emotional states I felt she was experiencing: Star of Bethlehem for her deep grief; Mimulus for her fear of being alone; Larch for her lack of self-confidence on making it on her own; Willow for her resentment towards her husband for leaving her; Walnut for the state of transition; Honeysuckle for clinging to the past and Sweet Chestnut for the deep depression she was in. I explained what each flower essence addressed, asking if she related to these states and was willing to be involved in this self-help treatment. She agreed with my recommendations. I asked her to call me in four to six weeks to follow up on her progress.

Barbara later called as requested and reported that she was doing much better since taking the flower essences.

Her depression and grief had eased a great deal, she felt less fearful and more confident in her ability to manage her life, and the feelings of resentment towards her husband were not as strong. She seemed surprised at how helpful the flower essences had been. She remarked that she didn't exactly understand how they worked yet, she was experiencing great relief. I felt she should continue with these original seven for another month or two, and then we'd speak again to determine if any changes would be indicated. Barbara agreed.

When we spoke two months later, Barbara was doing even better. She had been taking the flower essences for almost four months now and some changes were indicated. She felt she was over her issue of resentment towards her husband and was no longer living in the past. Her deep depression had lifted although feelings of grief still surfaced from time to time. She decided it was time to drop Willow, Sweet Chestnut, and Honeysuckle but still felt the need for Star of Bethlehem, Larch, and Mimulus. I felt she was well on her way to recovery from the emotional devastation of her husband's death.

(Note: In cases of divorce, also experienced as a deep loss for some, many of the above flower essences would also be extremely helpful. Many of the emotional states that are felt are quite similar.)

John, a twenty-five year old, had seen me in the past concerning his issue of breaking free from a domineering father. He was making good progress with this, having moved away from home, when a major crisis erupted in his life. The company he was working for was downsizing, and he had lost his job. He was quite depressed as well as concerned over how he would support himself. He felt going back home would negate the progress he had made with his father. His fear and anxiety were overwhelming and he felt discouraged. After going over his present issues together, the following flower essences were suggested for John's current state of emotional stress: Walnut, which was originally recommended for helping him break away from the dominance of his father. It seemed this issue wasn't completely released yet. Walnut would also assist now with this period of transition. Wild Oat would be helpful for a possible new life direction; Mimulus for his fear; Gentian for his discouragement and feelings of setbacks taking place in his life; and Rescue Remedy, for his state of general anxiety (Rock Rose, one of the flower essences in Rescue, assists in cases of terror and panic, and John was in a panic state; Impatiens assists in easing impatience, which John was certainly experiencing with finding another job as quickly as possible). John related to the indications of the suggested flower essences, and without hesitation agreed to try them. As he had already experienced success with the Bach flowers, he was more than willing to do so for his current situation.

I saw John some six weeks later and he seemed like another person. Many of the negative emotional states he had experienced after losing his job had abated. He was now attending school at night for a master's degree. He realized he needed to further his education to work in a field he really loved. Meanwhile, he found another job, although only temporary, in order to secure the funds to continue with his schooling and support himself. He felt he had a new future to look forward to. He no longer felt discouraged and saw the loss of his job in a new light. It provided him with the opportunity of making some changes he would not have had the courage to do before. We both agreed that he didn't need Wild Oat, nor Gentian or Rescue, as he had found his direction, was no longer discouraged, nor was he dealing with constant anxiety. He wanted to continue with Walnut and Mimulus, and Larch was now added, as he felt his self-esteem needed a boost in regard to finishing his master's degree.

There are other common life situations that may be stressful at times. I refer to marriage, becoming a parent, moving to a new home, and a change in career by choice, …as several examples. As we all know from personal experience, life is filled with change—life itself being a cycle of maturation. Change may be experienced as either positive or negative. Yet, regardless of how change is seen, there is always stress involved, with fear of the unknown assailing most of us.

MARRIAGE

The Bach Flowers can be incredibly helpful in assisting us through whatever changes we may go through, by releasing stress and emotional issues that may arise during these times. When getting married, most feel some apprehension, indicating Mimulus. Marriage is a time of transition. For this, Walnut is also indicated. And often, feelings of overconcern and worry for the new partner crop up, indicating Red Chestnut. New brides and grooms may feel overwhelmed as well, with the added responsibilities that marriage presents, and Elm may be indicated.

BIRTH OF A CHILD

The birth of a first child, although usually a joyous time for most of us, may also be a time of stress emotionally. Again, Walnut is indicated, with the transition from couple to family, and the adjustment to this major change in their lives. Elm may also be indicated, as many a new mother and/or father feel overwhelmed by this added responsibility. Fear of being a good parent, as well as lacking self-confidence in raising a child may come up, indicating Mimulus and Larch. Overconcern and worry for the health and safety of the baby may also be an issue, indicating Red Chestnut. And many times, the father may feel resentment over all the love and attention his wife now gives their offspring. He may feel somewhat neglected, indicating Willow.

MOVING

When a move comes up, even a planned one, this change can still bring stress. Of course, Walnut is always indicated, to help in breaking the old links to the past. Nostalgia and homesickness for the old home sweet home can be treated with Honeysuckle. With packing and unpacking and feeling overwhelmed by all the work still to do, Elm is indicated.

CHANGING CAREERS

Even by choice, a career change is always an anxious time. For fear of failure, Mimulus is indicated. Wild Oat may be indicated if there is uncertainty over career direction. Larch may be needed for lack of self-esteem and not feeling up to the challenge. Walnut is always indicated for any major change in life, to ease transitions.

RETIREMENT

Retirement, as well as aging, can be a stressful time. This is another major time of transition, and Walnut is once again indicated. Wild Oat is another consideration when these individuals feel they no longer have any purpose in life, or possibly even Wild Rose, if apathy sets in. Star of Bethlehem may be indicated, if feelings of grief and loss arise when the person feels forced to retire, as well as the need for Willow, for resentment. Honeysuckle may also be indicated for living too much in past memories, that prevent opening up to the opportunities life now presents. And Mimulus may also be indicated, when there is fear of no longer bringing home a salary and of loss of health.

As before, the common life scenarios just presented are illustrations of some of the many different emotional states that can come up during such experiences. Not everyone will experience them in the same way, nor have the need of the same flower essences. These situations have been generalized, to give you a deeper understanding of the various negative emotional states possible under such conditions and which of the 38 flower essences address them. Similar situations as described above now follow.

Case Histories:

Sally, a new mother, was having a problem in adjusting to the birth of her first child. She reported feelings of constant worry over the infant's well-being and was also feeling extremely overwhelmed with its continual care. She was in a state of exhaustion from lack of sleep when I saw her. She also expressed fear of not being a good enough mother, that she would hurt the child emotionally in some way. It seemed she also lacked confidence in her ability to care for her baby adequately. She was filled with anxiety and quite upset. After listening to Sally's plight, the following flower essences were suggested: Red Chestnut for overconcern; Elm for feeling overwhelmed; Olive for her extreme exhaustion; Mimulus for her fears of not being an adequate mother; Larch for lack of self-confidence in her role of mother; and Rescue Remedy for her extreme state of anxiety. Sally agreed with my evaluation of her emotional state, and was willing to try the recommended flower essences. She would call me in four weeks for a progress report. I heard from Sally within three weeks! The flower essences were already making a difference, and she couldn't wait to share her news. The extreme anxiety had totally disappeared, and her fear was lessening. She was also feeling more self-confident in her new role as a mother. Her overconcern was also easing up. Although she was still exhausted, it wasn't as extreme as before. She was still feeling overwhelmed however. Sally felt she no longer needed Rescue Remedy on a daily basis, nor Red Chestnut. She did feel the need to continue with Elm, Olive, Larch, and Mimulus for a while longer.

Tom had just retired when he came to see me. His wife Nancy was a client of mine, and when she realized Tom was in an emotional crisis, she asked if he would try the flower essences. He was experiencing a mild depression and appeared listless, withdrawing into himself. When we talked, he expressed sorrow over the loss of his youth, stating that he didn't know what he'd do with the rest of his life. There wasn't anything he felt he could do, and he seemed to long for the "good old days." After hearing his words, I suggested the following flower essences: Walnut for his state of transition; Wild Oat to bring a new path into view; Wild Rose for his sense of apathy and resignation; Star of Bethlehem for his sense of loss, and Honeysuckle, as it seemed he was stuck in the past. Tom related to the indications of these flower essences, and agreed to using them. I would speak with him in four weeks.

When we again spoke, Tom was no longer listless. He told me that he had taken up golf, something he had always wanted to learn, but never before had the time. He remarked that he was a bit surprised at his change in mood over the last few weeks. He had taken his retirement harder than he thought he would. He said it made him feel that his life was over. He now realized that although he was "getting on in years," he was still strong and healthy. And he now had the time to do many things that his work schedule had previously prevented. I noticed a complete change in Tom's energy. We went over the flower essences he had been taking, to determine if any changes were indicated. He no longer felt the need for Wild Rose. He said he was now taking his life back and was grateful for his change in attitude. He decided he'd continue with Honeysuckle, Star of Bethlehem, Walnut, and Wild Oat for a while longer however, as he was still experiencing feelings of nostalgia, loss, stress in adjusting to the life change, and he was still a bit uncertain as to what he wanted to do with the rest of his life. He also told me that although he knew the flower essences really helped his wife Nancy, he really didn't think they'd work for him.

Bach Flowers for Women's Issues

I feel it important to now focus on certain issues that pertain to women alone—issues that are not common to men. These issues can embrace not only the unique biological factors that at times put women at the mercy of their hormones, such as with PMS, pregnancy, childbirth, and menopause, but the mental challenges women also face in fully actualizing their own potential in what is still considered a "man's world." Although women have been slowly gaining ground in obtaining the same rights that men have, regretfully, true equality has not as yet been reached. While changes are indeed taking place, the effects of male chauvinism continue to be felt, with women struggling to take their rightful place beside their male cohorts. Lamentably, women are still seen by some men as inferior.

The movie *Tootsie*, starring Dustin Hoffman, attempted to bring to greater awareness the unfairness that women face in our society with the sexist attitudes of men that continue to prevail. While pretending to be a woman, Tootsie was faced with situations in which her worth as a female was disregarded, as well as being disrespected by men. For the first time in his life, he could relate to what it felt like in being a woman. He experienced this inequality firsthand. And it made him angry. Unfortunately, many women have to deal with what Tootsie did. The once familiar roles of women are expanding with issues of self-worth, respect, and a sense of personal accomplishment going beyond the roles of wife and mother.

The confusion surrounding a woman's role in today's changing world is a cause of emotional stress for many women. They often find themselves caught up in not only being wives and mothers, but taking on the added load of careers. "Super Mom" has become a term applied to more and more women, and the pressure that women find themselves under is not so easily dealt with. Once considered primarily male concerns, heart disease and other stress-related illnesses are now on the rise in women.

Some of the possible challenging situations that many women may have to deal with, and the many Bach Flowers that can bring balance to the negative emotional states and stress produced by these experiences are now explored.

ABUSIVE RELATIONSHIPS

Self-esteem is usually at the heart of this situation, with many women seeing themselves as helpless victims of male dominance. Often, these women were emotionally or physically abused as children, creating feelings of little self-worth. If there was no actual personal abuse, most likely they were privy to the abuse of their mothers. It then seems natural to accept abuse from male partners later on in their own relationships.

For women caught up in abusive relationships, the following flower essences are often indicated: Agrimony for denial; Centaury for being too passive and sacrificing one's own needs; Chestnut Bud for not learning from the past; Gorse for hopelessness; Larch for lack of self-worth; Mimulus for fear; Pine for guilt and feeling somehow deserving of abusive treatment; Star of Bethlehem for grief and trauma; Walnut to help break the link with the past and free oneself from an abusive partner; Wild Rose for resignation that nothing can be done to change the situation; and Holly for rage and hatred.

INCEST AND RAPE

These reprehensible acts can totally disempower a woman. The effects can be felt for her entire life with the damage to her sense of dignity and self-worth possibly scarring her forever. In our society, in cases of rape, there is still the lingering inclination to blame the woman, creating deep feelings of guilt and shame that somehow she brought it on herself. With incest, the young female is taught to see this act as one of receiving love from the adult male, creating great sexual confusion as well as guilt and shame.

For women who have been victims of incest or rape, the following flower essences are often indicated: Star of Bethlehem for grief and trauma; Crab Apple for feelings of shame and disgust, and feeling unclean; Gorse or Sweet Chestnut for hopelessness or deep anguish; Holly for rage and hatred; Pine for self-blame; White Chestnut for constant unwanted thoughts; Mimulus or Rock Rose for fear or terror; and Olive for emotional exhaustion.

ANOREXIA/BULIMIA

Eating disorders are much more common and prevalent in women. In our culture, there is so much emphasis placed on a woman's body, with Hollywood and Barbie dictating a quite unrealistic ideal for most women. Unfortunately, many women allow themselves to be taken in by this projection and hurt themselves in the process.

For women who suffer from eating disorders, among these anorexia and/or bulimia, the following flower essences are often indicated: Agrimony for their silent torment; Cherry Plum for loss of control expressed in their compulsive-obsessive behavior; Chestnut Bud for not learning from the past; Crab Apple for self-disgust; Gorse for hopelessness; Olive for exhaustion from gravely depleting the body; Larch for lack of self-worth; Mimulus for fear of obesity; Pine for not being "good enough"; White Chestnut for constant obsessive thoughts; and Walnut to withstand the influences of others.

PREGNANCY

For most women, pregnancy is embraced as a joyful time. However, this time in a woman's life can be wrought with great emotional fluctuation created by the hormonal shifts taking place in her body, affecting sleep, energy level, and greater emotional sensitivity. During this very special time in a woman's life, the following flower essences are often indicated.

1st Trimester

Hornbeam for loss of vitality; Rescue Remedy for morning sickness; Mimulus for fear; Scleranthus for hormone imbalances; Willow for resentment, in cases where the pregnancy is unplanned; Red Chestnut for fear of the baby's welfare; White Chestnut for an inability to sleep; and Walnut for this time of transition.

2nd Trimester

It is recommended to continue with Scleranthus and Walnut. Rsecue and Hornbeam may no longer be needed once into the fourth month, as nausea and fatigue usually abate. Many of the others suggested may also not be needed once into the 2nd trimester.

3rd Trimester

By the seventh month, Beech may be needed for supersensitivity to others; the indications for Elm may now come up—feeling overwhelmed at the prospect of having a baby; Impatiens may be also needed, especially in the ninth month, as the due date creeps up along with feelings of impatience; Crab Apple will probably be needed now, to help deal with body image in the final stages of pregnancy; a need for Mimulus may again be evident, with fear of going through the birthing process now developing; Red Chestnut, as well, may be needed for overconcern of safety for the baby; it is suggested that Walnut be continued throughout pregnancy; and the need for Rescue Remedy may also become evident now, with feelings of general anxiety and nervousness over giving birth.

During the Birth Process

It is highly suggested to make up a dilution bottle of the following flower essences to assist with the emotional ups and downs while giving birth. And don't wait for the last minute to prepare your bottle! Add Rescue Remedy, Olive, Elm, Beech, and Walnut as previously directed. This combination will be of great help during delivery. Remember—the flower essences may be taken as often as needed, without concern of overdosing or harming mother or the baby in any way. In fact, the baby will be also greatly assisted in its birthing process.

After Birth

The flower essences recommended after giving birth are: Olive for total exhaustion; Red Chestnut for overconcern for the infant; Elm and Larch for feeling overwhelmed, and lacking confidence in the new role of mother; Mustard for postpartum depression; Walnut to be continued in this state of transition of becoming a mother; and possibly Mimulus for fear of not adequately caring for the baby.

PMS (PREMENSTRUAL SYNDROME)

Many women experience emotional ups and downs and sometimes physical symptoms such as tender breasts and bloating just prior to their monthly period, due to hormonal changes in their bodies. The flower essences suggested for most women troubled by PMS are: Rescue Remedy for general tension and feelings of anxiety; Scleranthus for mood swings; Beech for hypercriticalness; Willow for feelings of resentment; Mustard for depression from no apparent cause; Hornbeam for feeling fatigued; and possibly Crab Apple for feeling unclean as bleeding begins.

Women who experience PMS may want to take some of the above mentioned flower essences (take only those which relate to the emotional discomfort you are feeling) just during this time. If you are already using other flower essences for current emotional issues in your life, simply stop these for a few days and substitute the flower essences needed for the stress caused from PMS. Once your period is over, resume using your original combination.

MENOPAUSE

This is a time in life that can be particularly challenging for many women—and a time of possible deep fear. In our youth-oriented culture, aging is unfortunately seen as something to dread, and even more so for women. We only have to look at the movie industry where leading men continue in these roles far into their senior years (as did Cary Grant and Clark Gable, for example), while leading women are very quickly given character roles once their prime is considered over. As men age, they become "distinguished," while women become "old ladies." Women seem to lose their value more quickly than do men. And sadly, menopause is viewed as the end of the productive years for women in more than one way. This can be one of the greatest emotionally challenging times that a woman may face. Especially in our patriarchal society, where menopause is saturated with negativity—instead of seen as an initiation into the Wise Woman years.

The flower essences suggested to help a woman through this time of major transition are: of course, number one, Walnut for transitions; Star of Bethlehem for grief and lost youth, and the possible trauma that is felt by some women; Mimulus for fear of aging, fear of illness, fear of abandonment, fear of loss of sexuality, etc.; Honeysuckle for longing for the good old days, and being stuck in the past; Scleranthus for mood swings caused by hormonal changes, as well as hot flashes, and one of the most highly recommended of the flower essences for this life passage; Gorse for hopelessness; Wild Rose for apathy and resignation; Willow for bitterness and resentment; Wild Oat for new life direction; and Rescue Remedy, which is extremely helpful for hot flashes, as well.

SELF-EMPOWERMENT

In the workplace, as well as in the home, women are no longer accepting unfair and unequal treatment, nor the unwarranted demands of others. Centaury enables a woman to recognize her own power, to be more assertive and not easily taken advantage of, both on the job, as well as in the home, when often exploited by family demands. Elm is wonderful for the Super Mom, relieving feelings of being overwhelmed, and helps prioritize what needs to be done. Oak is extremely helpful for the single mom who is raising a family and also working full time, and the career woman as well. Both can seem to struggle against formidable odds. Pine helps with women who are too hard on themselves, ever striving for perfection, as well as feeling guilty for the shortcomings of others. Vervain assists the overachiever, the woman who burns her candle at both ends and always feels keyed up, unable to relax. Mimulus releases fears of not succeeding or of success itself and instills courage. Gentian eases feelings of despair with setbacks and delays regarding career progress. Wild Oat assists in determining the correct path in life, and career direction if uncertain. Walnut helps with charting one's own course, and staying with it, despite what others may think. Willow assists with releasing resentment and bitterness when feelings of unfairness arise. And Larch is highly suggested for the woman who has low self-esteem, feels she won't succeed, and needs to be more confident that she can.

Please remember, these illustrations of possible women's issues and the flower essences that have been suggested for the probable emotional states that could arise are generalizations. Let us now look at some specific and individualized illustrations.

Case Histories:

Sherry had just been through an emotionally devastating divorce. She had lived with a man who had been emotionally and mentally abusive. She was in a state of severe depression when I saw her. There was deep-seated anger and rage, not only for her former husband but for herself as well for staying in an abusive relationship. She was having difficulty in functioning, with her depression preventing her from going on with her life. A rash had begun to develop on one of her legs which had become irritated by her constant scratching. Once I had a picture of Sherry's emotional state, I suggested the following flower essences to ease her stress: Star of Bethlehem for the emotional trauma, grief and loss she was experiencing; Walnut for the state of transition she was going through; Centaury for allowing another to take advantage of her, and not standing up for herself; Sweet Chestnut for the angst she was suffering from; both Willow and Holly for the bitterness and rage she expressed; and Wild Rose, as she appeared apathetic, her spirit seemingly all but gone. As I explained why I had chosen each, she was in agreement with my assessment. She would take these and call me in four weeks.

When I next spoke to Sherry, she advised that most of her depression had lifted, and she was beginning to make plans for a new life. She was still dealing with her feelings of bitterness and resentment, and felt there was a great deal yet left to process from all the years of abuse. Her feelings of grief and loss were less intense, although still present. What amazed her the most, however, was that the rash on her leg was healing. She stated that the flower essences really seemed to have made a difference in her emotional state. She would continue to take Star of Bethlehem, for her grief and loss; Willow and Holly for lingering feelings of bitterness and rage; Centaury, as she related to the personality type this flower essence represents, and wanted to be more self-assertive in the future. She would also continue with Walnut, as the transition was not over. She no longer felt the need to continue with Wild Rose or Sweet Chestnut, as she no longer felt apathetic or deeply depressed as before. Jointly, we agreed to add Wild Oat, as she had mentioned she wasn't quite sure of her new direction regarding work. She had been a housewife and mother for almost twenty years, not needing to work outside the home. She was now faced with finding a career. And since she was a bit apprehensive with both being on her own and going out to work, we also agreed that Mimulus was in order—for her fears.

Marge was beginning her change of life. She was sure her menopause had begun, as she was beginning to experience hot flashes and her period was two months late. It had only been a month since her symptoms began that Marge came to see me. She explained that she wasn't sleeping well, waking several times each night because of the hot flashes, and becoming exhausted. She was also becoming cranky and irritable and upset over her lack of patience. For the most part, she seemed to be accepting of this natural progression of her life and only concerned by her emotional discomfort that was causing a strain in her daily life. I suggested the following flower essences to ease Marge's situation: Rescue Remedy for the general stress and anxiety she was feeling (and Rescue contains Impatiens for irritability and tension, and Cherry Plum for feeling out of control), as well as to help with the hot flashes; Walnut for her state of transition; Scleranthus for the hormonal changes taking place; Beech for her temporary state of intolerance; and Olive for her exhaustion. I asked Marge to call me in four weeks for a follow-up. When she did, she reported that she was much calmer than before, less irritable and grouchy. She was also sleeping better. When she was awakened by a hot flash, she would just take some drops from her dilution bottle, and very quickly she'd able to go back to sleep. Her emotional distress was definitely easing. We then discussed which flower essences to continue with. She felt she would stay with all five for the present, and be in touch later on.

Elizabeth is a survivor of incest and child abuse. She was working with a therapist at the time that she came for a Bach consultation. This was initiated by recently becoming aware of early childhood memories that had been repressed, memories that were now causing her great emotional pain. When she heard about the Bach Flowers, she felt they might be another healing technique to work with, along with her therapy, in moving through a very distressful time. As we spoke, I could see how her childhood abuse had gravely affected her adult life. She had been in an abusive marriage and, when that finally ended, in several other abusive relationships. She had very little self-esteem and found it extremely difficult to take care of her own needs, always sacrificing them for others. She shared how hard it was to confront others when she felt unfairly treated. She could never let on that she was unhappy. Her early-life experiences had created a woman who saw herself a victim of others, undeserving of much, if any, consideration by others—whether it be in a relationship or at work. Elizabeth, however, was now ready to face her issues and desperately wanted to finally free herself from her past conditioning—from feeling and being a victim. The following flower essences were recommended: Agrimony for hiding her torments behind a brave front, as well as her inability to confront others; Star of Bethlehem for the trauma she had experienced as child and the grief now surfacing; Chestnut Bud for not falling into the old habit pattern of victim and reprogramming her old tapes; Centaury, the flower essence for those who allow others to take advantage of them, to give her the ability to now consider her own needs just as important as others; Walnut for protection against the influence of others, and to break the links from the past; Pine for her guilt feelings of "somehow it was her fault" for being abused; and Holly for her deep-seated feelings of rage and anger at what had taken place as a child. Elizabeth expressed great hope that the flower essences would be of help to her. She was to call me four weeks later.

When Elizabeth got back to me, as scheduled, she laughingly told me that her boss was beside himself! She was no longer the meek and mild woman he knew. She has begun to speak up for herself, to his consternation. She also shared that she's been having bouts with some depression, getting in touch with her childhood trauma. She understands, however, that this is part of her healing process and it needs to be released before her healing can be completed. I questioned if her emotional discomfort was manageable. She affirmed it was, and didn't feel the need to discontinue Star of Bethlehem (which is the one bringing up her feelings of deep grief, as well as releasing the emotional and physical trauma she suffered). She also didn't feel a need, at this time, to make any changes and said she wanted to continue with all the original flower essences as she feels they have been truly facilitating her healing process.

Bach Flowers for Children

It appears that the flower essences are even more effective with children! The baggage that most carry is a great deal lighter, as well as more short-lived, than that of adults, making for a faster reaction time in children. You will find that the Bach flowers are of great assistance in so many situations that children are subjected to. Many times, the emotional distress that affects our children goes unrecognized, as in a divorce. It is common, often, for both parents to be so caught up in their own emotional turmoil that they fail to notice the devastation that their children may be experiencing.

There are other times, as well, that parents may neglect to take into consideration the difficult emotional states their children may be going through. Fear of separation, even going to sleep at night, hyperactivity, the threat of a new baby, as well as learning disabilities are all very stressful and emotionally difficult situations that children may be faced with. The Bach Flowers can be of great assistance for your children's negative emotional states, as they are with your own.

DIVORCE

The Bach Flowers that are usually indicated to assist children with the emotional difficulties that come up during divorce are: Walnut for this difficult state of transition that children experience; Star of Bethlehem for the trauma and emotional sense of grief and loss; Scleranthus for when children are put in the position of choosing which parent they want to live with; Pine for the sense of guilt that many younger children feel that somehow they are to blame, that they were bad, and are now being punished. It's unfortunate that most young children are unable to understand the reasons for divorce, with their ability to discern or judge not yet well-developed, and magical thinking playing a large role in their world. Willow, for feelings of resentment towards one or both of their parents; Holly for anger and rage over the disruption of life and breakup of the family unit; Elm for feeling overwhelmed with the situation, and the many changes encountered; Honeysuckle for nostalgia and living in the past, and not accepting the current situation; Mimulus for feelings of fear that come up with the uncertainty of what now lies ahead; Gorse or Sweet Chestnut for depression, a feeling of hopelessness or extreme angst, and possibly Olive, if the trauma is particularly emotionally and/or physically depleting.

SEPARATION ANXIETY

The Bach Flowers that are usually indicated to assist those children who experience the emotional difficulties of separation are: Walnut to assist with the transition of separation from the parents (it is the "link breaker"); Honeysuckle to ease nostalgia and homesickness; Mimulus and Aspen for feelings of anxiety and foreboding; Rescue Remedy, the emergency combination for times of crisis and great anxiety (contains Rock Rose for terror and panic, and Star of Bethlehem for grief and loss); Chicory for overly possessive children; and Larch to boost self-confidence.

SLEEPING PROBLEMS

The Bach Flowers that are usually indicated to assist children with sleeping problems, often caused by fear of being left alone or threat of nightmares are: Rock Rose, Mimulus, and Aspen for terror, fear, and apprehension; Chicory for children who tend to be manipulative, and have a great need for attention; White Chestnut to help in relaxing the mind; Vervain for hyper children who are easily wound-up and find it hard to relax; and Rescue Remedy, the all-purpose crisis formula (which also contains Rock Rose for terror and panic).

HYPERACTIVITY

The Bach Flowers that are usually indicated to assist children who are hyperactive are: Vervain for the unusually active child who finds it hard to settle down; Impatiens for children who are keyed up and always in a rush; and Rescue Remedy itself is very helpful in bringing about a state of calm and relaxation once again.

ALLERGIES

There are two flower essences that are especially helpful with allergies—Walnut and Crab Apple. Walnut is a protection against the effects of outside influences. Pollen is certainly an outside influence. And Crab Apple is a cleanser for the system.

Children are not alone in suffering from the effects of allergies. I recently had the most amazing experience with Walnut at one of the Bach Seminars I present countrywide. My assistant for this seminar had advised me that she didn't know if she'd be able to work with me the whole weekend.

She had an extreme sensitivity towards environmental pollution, as well as being highly allergic to many substances. She hadn't been able to sleep in hotels. This would be her first attempt in several years. Although she had tried many different types of medication, nothing seemed to help. Without giving it much thought, I asked her if she'd like to try Walnut, explaining how effective it has been for allergy relief. As I always travel with the complete set of the Bach Flowers, I was able to make a dilution bottle for her on the spot. She was agreeable to giving it a try, and took Walnut throughout the day. When I saw her the next morning, she rushed over in great excitement and said to me, "It's a miracle! I was able to sleep undisturbed last night. I had no allergic reactions. Nothing has helped me before. I am amazed!" I was also amazed. I had never seen the flower essences work so quickly before (excluding Rescue Remedy, of course). We have since kept in touch, and her allergic reactions seem to be a thing of the past.

SIBLING RIVALRY

The Bach Flower Essences that are usually indicated to assist children who experience difficulty relating with other children in the family, whether it be the birth of a new brother or sister that threatens their position, or sibling rivalry itself, are: Walnut for the transition of no longer being the only child; Willow for feelings of resentment towards the sibling; Vine for bossy and aggressive children who always need to be in charge and have their way; Cherry Plum for the loss of temper, poor impulse control, and physical aggression; Chestnut Bud for the child who does not learn from past behavior; Holly for the child who has feelings of anger and rage, as well as envy and jealousy; and Larch for a poor self-image and lack of self-esteem. Many children with issues of sibling rivalry have feelings of inferiority, as well as jealousy, that are masked by their aggressive behavior.

LEARNING DISABILITIES

There are many issues that arise with children who have special problems. They are extremely sensitive little souls who realize they are different from other children. Many times this perceived difference brings on deep feelings of low self-esteem and possible depression. Limitations in learning can also cause frustration, guilt, and anger, as well as apathy.

The Bach Flower Essences that are usually indicated to assist children with learning disabilities are: Larch for low self-esteem, feeling inferior; Clematis and White Chestnut, as many are caught up in daydreaming and not in the present moment, seeming to be inattentive and forgetful, as well as unable to concentrate and focus. These two flower essences are excellent for grounding and concentration: Wild Rose for the child who becomes apathetic, appears listless, and seems to have given up; Chestnut Bud, which is helpful for learning from past mistakes, learning new lessons, and decreasing forgetfulness; Gentian for the despair caused by setbacks and delays that come with their progress (two steps forward, one step backward); Gorse and Sweet Chestnut may be indicated for deeper depression (feelings of hopelessness or extreme anguish); Agrimony for denial, concealing painful feelings from themselves and others (this can create a state of restlessness); Centaury, as many of these children allow themselves to be exploited and bullied by other children; Walnut for children easily influenced by other children or affected by their cruelty; Pine for feelings of guilt and self-blame; and Impatiens for tension, frustration, and impatience with themselves for not accomplishing tasks as easily as other children. It is common that many children with learning disabilities also suffer from hyperactivity. Several of the already noted flower essences indicated for this state may be applicable as well.

BEHAVIOR PROBLEMS

There are many other situations in which the flower essences can be of great assistance in treating unwanted or troubling behaviors in children: Vine for the child who is a bully and refuses to listen to authority; Cherry Plum for the child who has poor impulse control, is aggressive, and physically acts out, including temper tantrums; Mimulus for the shy, timid, and fearful child; Chicory for the child who is demanding and in need of constant attention; Walnut for transitions and changes, which are usually uncomfortable and create issues of adjustment—as when teething, starting school, puberty, moving, etc.; Mimulus and Cherry Plum have also been effective with bedwetting, addressing the emotional issues of fear and loss of control; Larch and Centaury for low self-esteem and allowing others to victimize them; and Aspen for hypersensitivity.

As before, the above illustrations are but some of the many different situations with their corresponding negative emotional states that may come up with children. Not all will experience them in the same way, nor have need of the same flower essences, nor are these states described definitive. Here are more specific and individualized illustrations presented for your future practice and use.

Case Histories:

Tina's mom was beside herself in relieving her five-year-old daughter's constant nightmares and resultant bedtime anxiety. Tina would awaken several times a week, screaming in terror. It had escalated to the point that Tina would no longer sleep alone. Tina's terror was now also causing a strain on the whole family. Her mother finally called for help. The flower essences we selected to help Tina over her fright and terror were: Rescue Remedy for her general state of anxiety (and Rescue contains Rock Rose for panic and terror, specifically); Mimulus and Aspen for her fear and apprehension; and Chicory for her recent possessive and clinging behavior. Tina was to be given this combination at least four times daily, and especially before going to bed. We also felt it best, for the first few nights, to allow Tina to sleep with her mom. Once the nightmares began to subside, Tina would again sleep in her own bed. Within the first week, the nightmares began to ease. By the end of the second week, they had just about stopped. Tina was no longer in a state of panic at bedtime, and was now able to stay in her own bed. Whatever had produced her nightmares seemed released. It was agreed to continue with these flower essences for another month. Once discontinued, if the nightmares should begin again, both Tina and her mom knew what to do.

Timmy was a bright five-year-old who was very attached to his mom. He would become quite upset whenever she left him with anyone. The situation worsened when, for the first time, he was to start school. While waiting for the school bus, he would begin to cry, and when it was time to get on, still crying, he would cling to his mother in panic. This was not only a stressful situation for Timmy, but for his distraught mother. As she had been using the Bach Flowers herself, she felt they would also be helpful for her son. After describing the situation to me, we felt the following flower essences were indicated to help relieve Timmy's intense emotional state: Rescue Remedy for the emotional crisis precipitated by going to school; Mimulus and Aspen for his extreme fear and apprehension; Honeysuckle for the separation anxiety he was feeling; and Walnut for this stage of transition with beginning school. It was also suggested that Timmy's mom add some Red Chestnut to her dilution bottle to ease her worry and concern for Timmy's current plight, as this was a difficult time for both of them. Little by little, as each day passed, Timmy was less panic stricken. It took almost a month for Timmy to be totally adjusted to the change in his life and no longer exhibit any apprehension of fear when going off to school. After two months, the flower essences were discontinued, and as it turned out, no longer needed.

Jordan was five when he was diagnosed with minor learning disabilities. He had a very short attention span and was also somewhat hyperactive. It was recommended by the school that he be placed in a special class for a year or two to receive the extra help and attention needed for him to catch up with his peers. Although Jordan had learning disabilities, he was aware enough to realize that something was wrong with him, and that he was in a special class. This seemed to affect him greatly, and his self-esteem plummeted. I became familiar with Jordan when his mother called, deeply concerned over her son. At the age of seven, she told me, he was talking about not wanting to live anymore. She had immediately gotten him into therapy, but also felt the Bach Flowers were another avenue to try, as they had been so helpful with her emotional issues. After discussing Jordan's situation and his current emotional state, the following flower essences were selected: Larch for his low self-esteem; Gorse for his state of depression; Vervain for his hyperactivity; Clematis and White Chestnut for his inattentiveness and lack of focus; Willow for his feelings of resentment for being different, and Star of Bethlehem for the trauma he suffered (being teased by other children). As Jordan had been suffering from these emotions for almost two years, his response to the flower essences took almost two months. Although his progress was slow in the beginning, by the end of the second month his turn around had begun. His depression had disappeared, with his self-esteem rising. His school work was also improving. His mother and I felt it a good idea to continue with these same flower essences for a while longer.

Lisa had been an only child for four years when her baby brother was born. This became a traumatic event for Lisa, as she had been the little princess of the family, and now there was a prince! Her mother thought she had prepared her daughter for the appearance of her new brother, and was quite shocked at Lisa's behavior. She wanted no part of her brother, and seemed very resentful, as well as in need of more attention than ever before. And she began to exhibit regressive behavior, pretending she was also a baby. Of course, Lisa's mom was well aware of what was going on. Lisa was evidently jealous of her new baby brother, and experiencing difficulty in accepting the change in her life. Despite her awareness, Lisa's mom was quite concerned over the situation, and soon called to inquire about flower essences for Lisa. The following are those selected for Lisa's distressing feelings: Walnut for her transition from only child to sister; Willow for her feelings of resentment; Chicory for her need of attention and possessiveness of her mother; Star of Bethlehem for the trauma and grief of no longer being #1; and Larch for low self-esteem and self-confidence. Lisa began to respond almost immediately to the flower essences. Her neediness subsided, and she began to take an interest in her new baby brother. Her feelings of resentment seemed to be replaced by wanting to mother him instead. She took delight in helping to feed him and play with him. She no longer saw him as a threat to her position in the family. This was also helped by her parents' awareness, and they made a strong effort to make sure she received her share of love and attention as well. After four weeks, it was decided to discontinue all but Larch and Walnut to assist Lisa with her self-esteem, as well as moving through her transition.

The flower essences are chosen for children as they are for adults—by noting the stressful emotional states being expressed and the child's personality Type. These are your guides to the flower essence or combination of essences needed to address the current situation. The dosage is the same with children as with adults, and is administered four times daily. You may make a dilution bottle or place at least four drops of the concentrate into milk or fruit juice. A baby who is being breast-fed can also receive the effects of the flower essences when the mother is taking them herself. Also in regard to infants—it is highly recommended to give all newborns Star of Bethlehem (or Rescue Remedy, which contains Star of Bethlehem), for release of the birth trauma that all experience.

Bach Flowers for Animals and Plants

We love them dearly and we know they love us every bit as much. They're our pets, our beloved companions, and we do everything in our power to protect them and keep them safe.

In this final chapter we will now turn to treating animals and plants, as the Bach Flowers facilitate emotional healing for all of God's creatures. The healing vibrations contained in the flower essences are effective for restoring emotional balance and harmony in *all* living things—from the Human to the Animal, as well as to the Plant Kingdom. And as with children, the Bach Flowers bring relief to animals and plants in a much shorter time.

One may wonder, "How do I determine which flower essences are needed by my pet? I can't communicate with them!" This is true. However, by being empathetic to their moods and possible emotional distress—and we all have this ability—we can get a pretty good feeling as to what they may be suffering. As all of us who have animals already know and don't need to be convinced of, our pets certainly have emotions. We know when they are happy or when they are distressed.

To determine which of the flower essences may be needed for particular crisis situations that our pets may be experiencing, we need to put ourselves in their shoes, so to speak. What would *you* be feeling if you were in the same situation? It most likely is the same for your cat or dog, or whatever other animal is sharing your life. And many times, when you are going through a particularly difficult period emotionally, your pet will be experiencing the same stressful state(s) that you are. It's also reassuring to know that a wrong selection cannot hurt your pet, nor are there any side-effects.

The following illustrations of many of the possible stressful states that animals may face are now provided to give you an understanding in selecting the appropriate flower essences that treat these states:

Agrimony assists with the torment that many animals face when a wound or injury is slow to heal.

Aspen is a great help with very nervous and easily frightened animals.

Centaury aids the runt of the litter who always seems to be pushed around by its bigger brothers and sisters.

Cherry Plum is for the very aggressive animal who may threaten to bite and seems uncontrollable.

Chestnut Bud is excellent in training. It prevents the same mistakes being made over again.

Chicory assists with animals that demand a lot of attention, and also for those who are too possessive of their owners.

Clematis is helpful for the animal that is always sleeping.

Holly assists with animals who seem jealous, and is also good for nasty temperaments.

Larch is extremely effective for the animal who seems to lack self-esteem and is low in the pecking order.

Mimulus helps with fear, as with thunderstorms, for example, and is also for the very timid and shy animal.

Olive is extremely helpful after an illness or operation.

Rock Rose treats extreme panic and terror.

Star of Bethlehem is for any trauma, shock or grief an animal may experience. It is especially helpful with animals who have been victims of abuse.

Vervain, and also **Impatiens**, are very effective with high-strung, nervous animals.

Vine is used for the animal who won't accept authority, and also for the boss animal who dominates other animals it lives with.

Walnut is always indicated for any change taking place in an animal's life, such as a move, a new owner, a new pet introduced into the home, as well as a new child.

Water Violet is used with aloof animals who tend to be loners and is the personality Type for most cats.

Wild Rose is needed when an animal appears listless and apathetic.

Willow is excellent when feelings of resentment may crop up, as with a new pet or birth of a baby.

And the final selection—for all emergency crisis situations:

Rescue Remedy—When in doubt as to which flower essence may be needed, Rescue is always helpful in just about any situation that may arise for animals. I give my animals Rescue on a daily basis as a general balancer and de-stressor. And don't forget to give your pet some Rescue before a visit to the vet, which always produces great anxiety. You will be amazed at how Rescue eases your pet's panic attack.

The following illustrations are cases from my practice in which the Bach Flowers have been used with remarkable results with animals in distress. Know that the flower essences are not only a wonderful assistance in regard to maintaining general emotional well-being, but are also extremely effective in modifying behavioral problems.

Case Histories:

Rocky was adopted by the Smith family at about six weeks of age. He was a normal, healthy, friendly, and playful kitten. Several weeks later, the Smiths' two young sons left for camp. When they returned home at summer's end, dramatic changes in Rocky's personality abruptly took place. This once friendly, easy-going kitten had became a recluse, hiding under the bed and only coming out to eat dinner. This became his way of life. No one could go near him except Mr. or Mrs. Smith, and even with them he was extremely nervous. They had their suspicions that one of their sons had traumatized the kitten in some way, although they could never get either of them to fess up to any foul play. Rocky remained in his shocked and fearful state for over two years, until Mrs. Smith learned of the Bach Flowers. She was extremely encouraged and hopeful that they would help Rocky's plight. In discussing the case with them, we began the task of selecting the essences we felt were appropriate for his emotional condition—one dominated by extreme fear, suspicion, and terror. After carefully considering Rocky's emotional state, we selected the following six flower essences that addressed what we felt he was experiencing: Rock Rose, for extreme terror and panic; Mimulus, for fear; Aspen, for apprehension (as his fear was so extreme, we felt it best to touch all bases); Scleranthus, for emotional instability; Holly, for suspicion and mistrust; and Star of Bethlehem, for whatever shock and trauma that had caused the radical change in Rocky's behavior. Six weeks passed before any noticeable changes occurred, and when they did, they were dramatic. A turnabout in his behavior had begun. While Mrs. Smith's mother was visiting, Rocky actually came out from hiding, approached her, sashaying his way across the room, and let her pet him. He then went to the kitchen door, requesting to be let out. Mrs. Smith's mother commented to her, "I had forgotten you had that cat, haven't seen him in ages!" and proceeded to open the door for him. Mrs. Smith told me that she was in shock for the moment! This was the first time since Rocky's out-of-balance emotional condition had developed that he had appeared with unfamiliar people present. His new lease on life was initiated. Rocky no longer stayed in hiding under the bed, and except for one of the Smith boys (and this is a major clue as to which one may have traumatized him!), he no longer displays fear towards people. Rocky is now a happy, healthy, mostly well-adjusted cat. (Let's be honest, how many cats are totally well-adjusted!) Mr. Smith, who was a skeptic at first, was quite impressed with the change in Rocky; so much so that he now takes the flower essences himself.

A woman recently called concerned about her horse Baby. He had become apathetic and listless, and she was worried about his health. I suggested she give him Wild Rose for his seeming apathy and resignation. A few weeks later, she called me back to report that Baby was up and about, and back to his normal self.

I received another call from a man, someone I had helped in the past, and had recommended the use of Rescue

Remedy. He was calling to share a wonderful story in which Rescue had been extremely helpful. Recently, his colt Black Beauty had caught his hind leg in a fence and had cut some tendons. After first calling the vet, he then began to treat the colt every fifteen minutes with Rescue, as it would take a while for the vet to get to him. About an hour later the vet arrived and was amazed that he was able to stitch and dress the wound without a tranquilizer. The wound had to be treated and dressed for three months, and he continued using Rescue before each treatment to keep Beauty calm, as well as administering Rescue to the horse daily to assist his healing process.

Bobbi, a client of mine herself, called one day about her cat Angel, who wouldn't use the litter box. She certainly wasn't living up to her name! Angel would normally relieve herself outside the house. It became a problem, however, when she was unable to go out because of rain or snow. When this took place, she would use the bathroom rug instead of the litter box. Bobbi had tried numerous times to train Angel to use her box, to no avail. She felt this couldn't go on much longer. Bobbi was now turning to the flower essences before giving up her pet. Chestnut Bud was suggested, for failure to learn from past mistakes and repeating the same mistake many times over. This flower essence has been extremely effective in training many animals, as well as correcting any bad habits, like scratching on the furniture. I am happy to report that Angel is now using her litter box, and a good thing for her. She was on the verge of losing her home, and possibly her very life. Bobbi was quite amazed, as well as extremely grateful, at how helpful Chestnut Bud was and how quickly it worked. Within two days, Angel had been retrained. Bobbi was greatly relieved, as she deeply loved her cat, and had been distressed at the possibility of giving Angel up. I suggested she continue using Chestnut Bud for a while longer, and also to use Rescue Remedy everyday and always, as a general balancer.

The Bach Flowers help with all animals—even with birds and fish. I have had the personal experience of rescuing several birds that my cats, regrettably (for me!), brought home from time to time. They are lucky enough to still be alive thanks to Rescue Remedy. I have learned firsthand, many times over, why it's called the emergency first aid treatment. I place a few drops (I always make a dilution bottle because of the great amount of brandy in the concentrate, which makes it difficult for animals to accept) on their beaks and rub some on their heads. I then place them in a box I have filled with some grass and put them in a safe place. Every half hour I give another dose. As they recover, I make arrangements to bring them to a local bird sanctuary to complete their healing process. I'll never forget the time when one of my rescued baby birds, after seeming almost dead, hopped onto the edge of her box and sang her little heart out! I had put her in an upstairs bedroom safely away from her predator and had closed the door. Several hours later, I began to hear her chirping. When I went to check on her, I found her amazingly well. And Rescue Remedy even works with fish. A friend of mine has tropical fish that almost died. She was able to bring them around by placing several drops in their fish tank.

Sammy, my good friend Linda's dog and faithful companion for many years, suddenly refused to eat or drink. Linda became very concerned and called me for help with the Bach Flowers. I soon learned that Linda's cat—a playmate of Sammy—had died two days ago. These two animals had become inseparable friends. I strongly felt that Sammy was mourning the loss of his friend. With Rescue Remedy in hand, off I went to Linda's. Once there, we began treating the dog with Rescue. I had made a dilution bottle and continued giving him several drops every fifteen minutes. When I left, I told Linda to continue treating Sammy with the Rescue, and I'd call the next day to see how he was progressing. When I spoke to Linda the next morning, she said Sammy had eaten a bit, but was still languishing. I brought over Sweet Chestnut and Wild Rose to be added to Sammy's dilution bottle—for his anguish and listless state. After about two weeks on the flower essences, Sammy was his old self again. And Linda had also gotten another kitten as a new playmate for him.

Karen had two dogs, one from birth, Bo, and the other, Floyd, only recently adopted. She called one day, hoping the flower essences would help, relating the following situation to me. Bo had always been a timid dog, and not all that affectionate. Floyd, on the other hand, was quite possessive, and very jealous. He was forever picking on Bo and gave him no peace. The flower essences that were indicated for the emotional states of Bo and Floyd were: Mimulus for Bo's timidity, and Water Violet for his aloofness; Chicory for Floyd's possessiveness, Holly for his jealousy, and Vine for his domineering behavior. After about three weeks, Linda reported that changes had begun to take place in both dogs. Bo is much more affectionate and no longer cowers in the presence of Floyd, with the help of Water Violet and Mimulus. And Floyd has become much more tolerant of Bo, his domineering behavior and possessiveness slowly diminishing with the help of Holly, Vine, and Chicory. I suggested that these flower essences be continued for awhile longer. I also advised that it may be possible that Bo is a natural Mimulus Type, and that Floyd is a Vine Type. Both might do well to continue with these flower essences as their personality essences on a permanent basis.

Administering the flower essences to animals is as easy as placing a few drops of the concentrate in their drinking water or food—four drops of Rescue, and/or two drops of any of the other 38 flower essences that you have selected. And don't worry about your other pets who may not need the same essences and drink or eat from the same bowls. The flower essences will not affect them if they do not need them. Remember, a wrong selection does nothing. A dropper bottle dilution preparation may also be made to administer directly into the animal's mouth. The directions are the same for animals as for humans. It is suggested however, not to use alcohol as a preservative in your pet's dilution bottle. Its taste seems to be an unwelcome one for pets.

Seven flower essences is also the generally recommended limit for your pets, as with you. Larger animals (horses, etc.) can be given the flower essences with the aid of a large dosage syringe available from livestock supply companies. As with humans, the flower essences are administered four times daily. In cases of extreme stress or crisis, they may be given every fifteen minutes. And remember, there is no danger of overdosing. From my personal experience with my own pets, they seem to know that the flower essences are helping them, and easily accept taking them.

The Bach Flowers may also be used for plants, and are highly effective in many situations. Although plants may not appear to be very conscious or to have feelings, my understanding of this was radically changed by reading Peter Tompkins's book, *The Secret Life of Plants*, many years ago. According to Tompkins's information, plants actually respond to perilous circumstances, and possibly may experience feelings of fear as well as other stressful states.

This book describes an experiment that was done where electrodes were attached to a group of plants to see if it was possible to monitor electrical impulses produced by them in various situations. In one situation, one of the experimenters purposely killed one of the plants in the group. While this was taking place, unusual electrical activity was picked up. A day or so later, different individuals, including the perpetrator, would go into the room where the murder took place, while one of the researchers monitored any activity. When the experimenter who had done the deed entered the room, the needle went off the page!

This and various other experiments described in this book appear to point to the fact that plants, indeed, have consciousness—more than we would imagine. It would therefore seem beneficial, from what we know of the Bach Flowers, to make use of their efficacy with our plants as well. And from my personal experiences in doing so, as well as that of many others I know, this appears to be extremely helpful. The following are illustrations of generalized situations in which flower essences may be effectively used for plants.

Whenever transplanting, Rescue Remedy is recommended for the shock and trauma experienced from this procedure. For insect infestation, Crab Apple is highly recommended. When moving plants to another location, Walnut is suggested for this state of transition and change. For plants that have been attacked by a pet, Mimulus is the flower essence to use. When a plant appears drooping, some Hornbeam will perk it up. And for cut flowers, to assist in keeping them fresh longer, Rescue is also recommended.

I have been adding Rescue to cut flowers for years now, and they definitely keep longer. Once a month I spray some Rescue on all my house plants,. My plants are just thriving, all lush and vibrant. The following experience is presented now to give you a more specific illustration of the help available for plants with the use of the flower essences.

I recently had an occasion to see how incredible the flower essences are with plants in crisis. This past June, I had planted three azaleas in my front garden. After a few days, one of the new plants began to wilt and looked pretty pathetic. It looked like I might lose it. I quickly made up a combination in a bucket, using eight drops of each of the following flower essences: Rescue Remedy for the crisis situation (and it also contains Star of Bethlehem, for shock and trauma), Hornbeam and Olive for sapped vitality and major exhaustion, Wild Rose for its listless appearance, Walnut for just being transplanted and its state of transition, and Centaury, as it seemed quite weak. I first poured a bucketful around the base of the plant, and then every half hour I sprayed its wilted leaves. When I checked on it the next morning, it hadn't seemed to respond. I didn't give up, though, and continued to spray it throughout the day. The next morning, I could not believe my eyes. It had perked up and now was as strong and healthy looking as the other two just-planted azaleas. It was an incredible feeling to be able to bring the plant around again. At this writing, it is the end of August, and the azalea plant is absolutely thriving!

Afterword

"This system of treatment is the most perfect that has been given to mankind within living memory. It has the power to cure disease; and, in its simplicity, it may be used in the household.

It is its simplicity, combined with its all-healing effects, that is so wonderful.

No science, no knowledge is necessary, apart from the simple methods described herein; and they who will obtain the greatest benefit from this God-sent Gift will be those who keep it pure as it is; free from science, free from theories, for everything in Nature is simple.

There is little more to say, for the understanding mind will know all this, and may there be sufficient of those with understanding minds, unhampered by the trend of science, to use these Gifts of God for the relief and the blessing of those around them."

Dr. Edward Bach
The 12 Healers

We are on the verge of a paradigm shift in regard to healing. We are beginning to understand our personal responsibility for our health, and that we influence—directly or indirectly—our well-being on some level, by our attitudes and emotions. When these are negative, we now know we cause biological changes in our brain chemistry that adversely affect our health. If we can affect our health negatively, the good news is that we can also affect our health *positively*. The Bach Flowers are one healing modality that works to this end, with the restoration of emotional balance and harmony to our system, thus preventing the manifestation of disease. We are slowly moving beyond traditional medicine. We are discovering new options in health care, and with these options, empowering ourselves to be our own healers, for this is where healing truly begins, *within ourselves.*

I created this book as a resource and guide for you in your application and practice of the Bach Flowers—one that may be referred to any time you feel the need to change the flower essences you are taking—to assist you in your new selections. Use it not only for yourself but for others you may wish to help. I trust this information will facilitate your work with the flower essences so that you may also discover, as I have, their powerful yet gentle action in restoring balance and harmony to your body, mind, *and* spirit.

It has been my joy and pleasure, and an honor and privilege, in sharing with you Dr. Edward Bach's extraordinary self-help system. I am forever grateful to Dr. Bach for the gift of his flower essences and the transformation they have brought to my life. I am confident that you will feel the same as you go on to utilize them yourself. I invite you now to take charge of your own health and well-being—to discover for yourself this very special catalyst for personal growth and emotional healing.

Many blessings to you all...
Rachelle

"The action of these remedies is to raise our vibrations, and open our channels for reception of our Spiritual Self; to flood our natures with the particular virtue we need, and wash out from us the fault which is causing harm. They are able, like beautiful music, or any glorious uplifting thing which gives us inspiration, to raise our very natures, and bring us nearer to our Souls: and by that very act, to bring us peace, and relieve our sufferings. They cure, not by attacking disease, but by flooding our bodies with the beautiful vibrations of our Higher Nature, in the presence of which disease melts as snow in the sunshine."

Dr. Edward Bach
Ye Suffer From Yourselves

PERMISSIONS

Recommended Reading and Resources

BOOKS

The Bach Flower Remedies, Edward Bach, MD, & F. J. Wheeler, MD. Keats Publishing Co.

The Original Writings of Edward Bach, Judy Howard & John Ramsell. The C. W. Daniel Company, Ltd.

The Medical Discoveries of Edward Bach, Physician, Nora Weeks, The C. W. Daniel Company, Ltd.

Handbook of the Bach Flower Remedies, Philip M. Chancellor, (Editor). Keats Publishing Co.

Bach Flower Remedies Step by Step, Judy Howard. C.W. Daniel Company, Ltd.

BFR Questions & Answers, John Ramsell. The C. W. Daniel Company, Ltd.

Bach Flower Remedies for Women, Judy Howard. C.W. Daniel Company, Ltd.

Bach Flower Remedies for Men, Stefan Ball. C.W. Daniel Company, Ltd.

Growing Up with Bach Flower Remedies, Judy Howard. C.W. Daniel Company, Ltd.

VIDEOS

* *The Light That Never Goes Out*
* *Bach Flower Remedies, A Further Understanding*

If you are unable to locate any of the above in your local bookstores, you may order by calling Nelson Bach, USA 1-800-314-2224

BACH FLOWER ESSENCE EDUCATIONAL SEMINARS

A. Nelson & Co. Ltd., in conjunction with the Edward Bach Centre in England, is currently presenting outstanding Seminars on the Bach Flower Essences countrywide. Call 1-800-314-BACH for further information regarding the Seminar Schedule for the current dates and locations throughout the United States.

BACH FLOWER ESSENCE AUDIO CASSETTES

Produced and Studio Recorded by Rachelle Hasnas

* *The 39 "Healers" of Dr. Edward Bach*	$11.95
* *Affirmations, Enhancing Bach Flower Therapy*	$11.95

Audio cassettes may be purchased directly from Rachelle. To order, mail your Check or Money Order in the amount indicated above, plus an additional $3 for shipping and handling, to:

Rachelle Hasnas
1063 Tottenham Lane
Virginia Beach, VA 23454

The Bach Flower Essences are available in most heath food stores. If yours does not carry them, they may be ordered directly from the distributor, Nelson Bach, USA, by calling 1-800-314-2224.

Other pocket guides from The Crossing Press

Pocket Guide to The 12-Steps
By Kathleen S.
$6.95 • Paper • ISBN 0-89594-864-8

Pocket Guide to Shamanism
By Tom Cowan
$6.95 • Paper • ISBN 0-89594-845-1

Pocket to Self Hypnosis
By Adam Burke
$6.95 • Paper • ISBN 0-89594-824-9

Pocket Guide to Ayurvedic Healing
By Candis Cantin Packard
$6.95 • Paper • ISBN 0-89594-764-1

Pocket Herbal Reference Guide
By Debra Nuzzi
$6.95 • Paper • ISBN 0-89594-568-1

Pocket Guide to Numerology
By Alan Oken
$6.95 • Paper • ISBN 0-89594-826-5

Pocket Guide to the Tarot
By Alan Oken
$6.95 • Paper • 0-89594-822-2

Please look for these books at your local bookstore or order from
The Crossing Press, P.O. Box 1048, Freedom, CA 95019.
Add $2.50 for the first book and 50¢ for each additional book.
Or call toll-free 800-777-1048 with your credit card order.